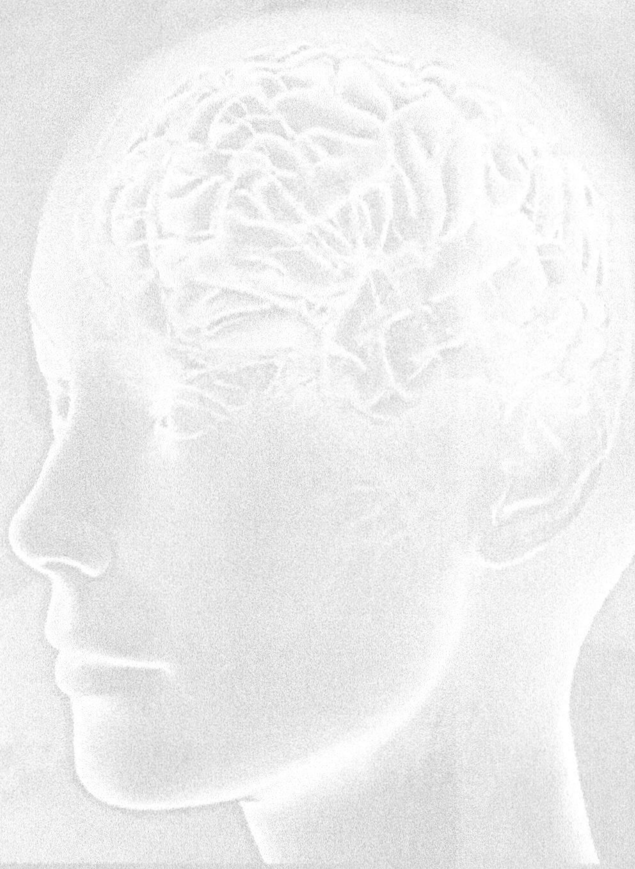

# AMYOTROPHIC LATERAL SCLEROSIS

# AMYOTROPHIC LATERAL SCLEROSIS

## Advances and Perspectives of Neuronanomedicine

Lina Machtoub
Yu Kasugai

Pan Stanford Publishing

*Published by*

Pan Stanford Publishing Pte. Ltd.
Penthouse Level, Suntec Tower 3
8 Temasek Boulevard
Singapore 038988

Email: editorial@panstanford.com
Web: www.panstanford.com

**British Library Cataloguing-in-Publication Data**
A catalogue record for this book is available from the British Library.

**Amyotrophic Lateral Sclerosis: Advances and Perspectives of Neuro-nanomedicine**



ISBN 978-981-4463-04-1 (Hardcover)
ISBN 978-981-4463-05-8 (eBook)

Printed in the USA

# Contents

*Preface* vii

**1 Clinical Features of Amyotrophic Lateral Sclerosis** **1**
1.1 What Is Amyotrophic Lateral Sclerosis? 1
1.2 ALS Signs and Symptoms 3
1.3 The Different Types of ALS 6
1.3.1 Familial ALS (Hereditary) 7
1.3.2 Familial ALS: Signs and Symptoms 13
1.3.3 How to Manage Familial ALS? 14
1.3.4 Sporadic ALS (Acquired) 14
1.3.5 Sporadic ALS: Signs and Symptoms 15
1.4 ALS: Clinical Case Studies 19

**2. Environmental Factors** **25**
2.1 What Environmental Factors Are Suspect in ALS? 25
2.2 Toxic Metals and Solvents 27
2.3 The Possible Effects of Exercise or Pesticides 28
2.4 Environmental Influences of Viruses 28
2.5 BMAA Neurotoxic Effects 29
2.6 Are Toxins in Seafood Causing ALS? 30

**3 Diagnostic Criteria of Amyotrophic Lateral Sclerosis** **35**
3.1 Steps in the Diagnosis of ALS 35
3.1.1 History and Physical Exam 37
3.1.2 Electrophysiology Studies 37
3.1.3 Radiology Studies 41
3.2 Electrophysiology in the Revised EEC 47
3.3 Nerve Conduction Studies 47
3.4 Clinical Features in the Diagnosis of ALS 48

3.5 Inconsistent Clinical Features 50
3.6 ALS Electrophysiological Features 51
3.7 ALS Neuroimaging Features 55

**4 Perspectives of Neuronanomedicine 59**
4.1 Nanomedicine and Neurological Disorders 59
4.2 CNS Neuroprotective Potentials 64
4.3 Nanocarriers and CNS-Targeted Drug Delivery 68
4.4 Applications Based on Cell-Mediated Drug Delivery 77
4.5 CNS Nano-Based Diagnostic Approaches 80
4.5.1 Proposed in vitro Nanodiagnostic Approaches 83
4.5.2 Proposed in vivo Nanodiagnostic Approaches 84
4.5.2.1 Nano-based optical imaging 86
4.5.2.2 SECARS microscopy 87
4.6 Inflammation and Neurodegeneration: Can We Measure Neuroprotection and Repair through Imaging Techniques? 88
4.7 Constraints in the Treatment of Neurodegenerative Diseases: Future Directions 91

**5 Novel Therapeutic Approaches 99**
5.1 Conventional Treatments for ALS 99
5.2 Occupational Therapy and Supportive Therapy 100
5.3 Cell Replacement Therapy and Future Challenges 102
5.4 Stem Cell Transplantation Therapy 113
5.5 Clinical Applications of Cell Transplant Therapy 116
5.6 Trials of Other Cell Sources for Stem Cell Therapy 119
5.7 Stem Cell Therapy: Clinical Trials 122
5.8 Induced Pluripotent Stem (iPS) Cell Therapy 124
5.9 Gene Therapy and Future Challenges 127

*List of Abbreviations* 143
*Index* 147

# Preface

Amyotrophic lateral sclerosis (ALS) is one of the most devastating motor system neurodegenerative diseases, causing around 10,000 deaths each year. The neuropathology of ALS, which leads to muscle weakness, is mostly confined to motor neurons in the cerebral cortex, motor nuclei of the brainstem, and anterior horns of the spinal cord.

The major goal in treating ALS, currently, is to recognize the onset of the disease early in order to initiate appropriate therapy and delay functional and cognitive losses. Upon the discovery of mutated SOD1 in ALS, many hypotheses have been proposed on how mutant SOD1 could cause neurodegeneration, including aberrant redox chemistry, mitochondrial damage, excitotoxicity, microglial activation and inflammation, as well as SOD1 aggregation. Recently, the implication of biocompatible nanotechnologies set the stage for an evolutionary leap in diagnostic imaging and therapy. In this scope, the book provides a comprehensive overview of the hypotheses and the molecular mechanisms associated with the inflammatory processes in motor neuron disorders and presents the latest research studies on ALS, highlighting the recent findings using newly developed imaging modalities and the innovative approaches of highly sensitive molecular imaging. In addition, by using recently developed surface-enhanced nanoimaging microscopy, the book offers new perspectives on neuroimaging and insights into early diagnosis and promising therapeutic strategies.

**Lina Machtoub and Yu Kasugai**
Universitätsklinik für Radiodiagnostik
Medizinische Universität Innsbruck
Anichstr.35, 6020 Innsbruck, Austria
May 2015

# Chapter 1

# Clinical Features of Amyotrophic Lateral Sclerosis

The aim of this chapter is to introduce some basic concepts about amyotrophic lateral sclerosis (ALS). We start by outlining the concepts of motor neuron diseases and the clinical features of ALS, and present some recent clinical case studies. This will act as a basis to understand the subsequent chapters.

## 1.1 What Is Amyotrophic Lateral Sclerosis?

Motor neuron disease, interchangeably known as amyotrophic lateral sclerosis (ALS), is a neurodegenerative disorder characterized by a progressive muscular paralysis reflecting degeneration of motor neurons in the primary motor cortex, brain stem, and spinal cord. The disease mainly affects patients between 50 and 70 years of age. ALS was originally described by the French physician Jean-Martin Charcot in the 1870s (Fig. 1.1). ALS is widely known as Lou Gehrig's disease, named after the famous baseball player Lou Gehrig, who died of ALS, and which confines star British physicist Stephen Hawking to the wheelchair (Fig. 1.2). ALS is universally fatal, with an average mortality of 5 years after onset.

*Amyotrophic Lateral Sclerosis: Advances and Perspectives of Neuronanomedicine*
Lina Machtoub and Yu Kasugai

ISBN 978-981-4463-04-1 (Hardcover), 978-981-4463-05-8 (eBook)
www.panstanford.com

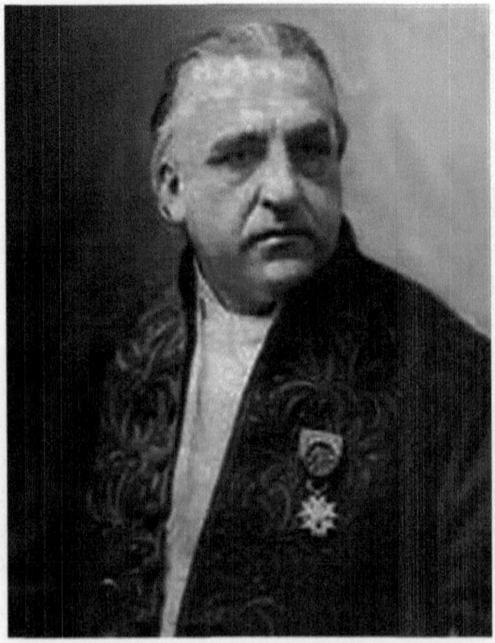

**Figure 1.1** Dr. Jean-Martin Charcot, who first described ALS in a publication in Paris (1869).

The phenotypic expression of ALS is highly heterogeneous and determined by four elements: (1) body region of onset, (2) relative mix of upper motor neuron (UMN) and lower motor neuron (LMN) involvement, (3) rate of progression, and (4) cognitive impairment. ALS causes progressive weakness, which may at first be mild and subtle, but becomes severe and eventually affects the breathing muscle machinery. This disease ultimately results in death. The onset of the disease is insidious, and symptoms may be disregarded by the patient for several weeks or months. The first physicians consulted are usually general practitioners, orthopedic surgeons, or rheumatologists and only rarely neurologists. Even in countries with well-developed healthcare systems, it takes a year on average before the diagnosis is made. Up to now the diagnosis of ALS is still a clinical one and electromyography (EMG) is the most important technical test to support the diagnosis. Laboratory tests

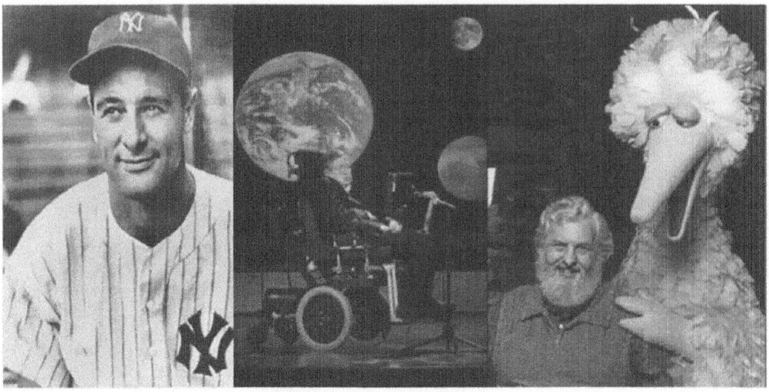

**Figure 1.2** Notable people affected with ALS: (left) Lou Gehrig, Stephen Hawking, and (right) Jon Stone.

and imaging, including MRI, do not yield diagnostically positive results, but are necessary to exclude other potentially better treatable diseases.

## 1.2 ALS Signs and Symptoms

The first symptoms of ALS may be so subtle that they are overlooked: like muscle twitching, cramping, stiffness, weakness, involuntary jerking movements, tremors, inability to control the bowels or the bladder, or inability to move or open the eyes completely. As the weakness in the limb muscles progresses, muscle tissue is lost (atrophy), and the arms and legs begin to look thinner. Speech may become slurred, and later chewing and swallowing become difficult. Individuals with this disorder lose their strength, the ability to walk, and use of their hands and arms. Breathing becomes difficult because the muscles of the respiratory system weaken. Most people with ALS die from respiratory failure (Fig. 1.3).

There have been numerous debates on whether the upper or the lower motor neuron is first affected by the disease process. Upper motor neuron signs are preserved or exaggerated tendon reflexes in the presence of muscle atrophy and weakness. The muscle tone may be increased corresponding to spasticity more in the lower than

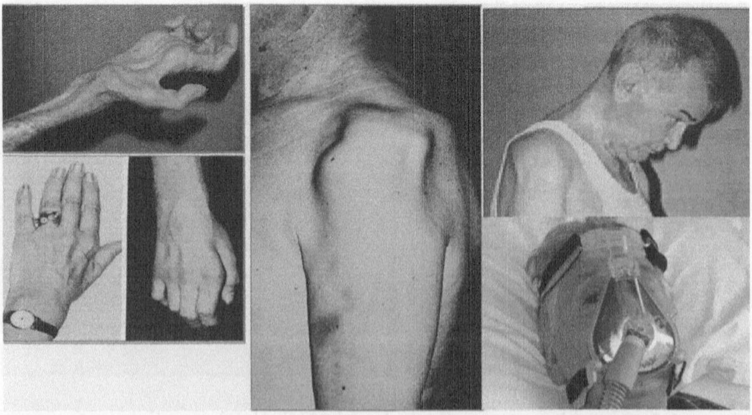

**Figure 1.3** The hallmark of ALS is muscle denervation and wasting. Noninvasive ventilation of a patient with ALS. Photos courtesy of Robert Brown, MD, Harvard Medical School, Massachusetts General Hospital. V. McGuire et al., *Neurology* 1996;47: 571–573.

the upper extremities. In about 30% of the cases a Babinski sign may be observed. Signs of corticobulbar involvement are increased masseter reflexes, pathological laughing, crying, and yawning, which are also called pseudobulbar affect. The manifestation of upper and lower motor neuron features usually begins focally and progresses to involve contiguous regions of the body with decreasing severity. Approximately two-thirds of cases start in the limbs and one-third in the bulbar group of muscles; only a very small percentage of them begin with respiratory muscle involvement. Many patients, however, do not show signs of the upper motor neuron in early stages of the disease. Signs of the lower motor neuron are muscle atrophy, weakness, and fasciculations. In early stages of the disease, patients frequently speak of clumsiness and not so often of weakness. The onset of ALS is usually focal and asymmetrical: in somewhat more than 30% of the cases in the upper extremities, in about one-third in the lower extremities, and in about 25% in the bulbar region. A special phenotype is the so-called flail arm syndrome with onset of muscle weakness in the proximal upper extremities, while the legs may be spared for a long time. The flail leg syndrome with onset of the symptoms in the proximal lower extremities is observed less

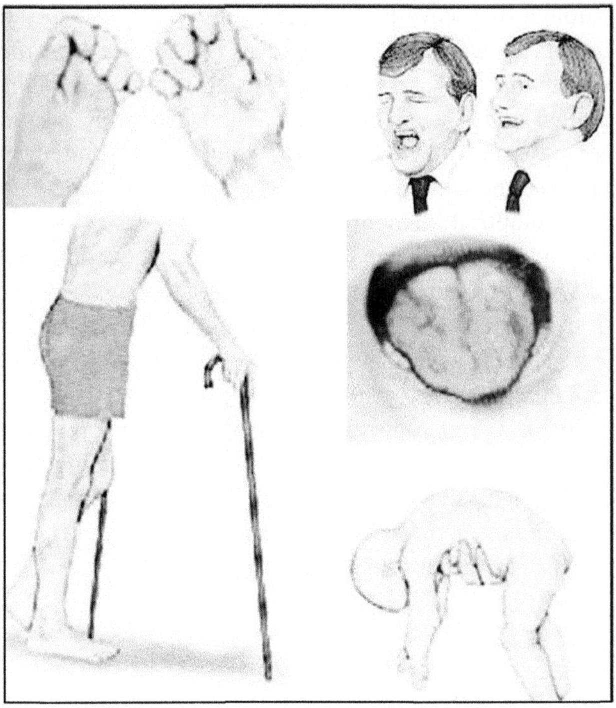

**Figure 1.4** Lesions of both first and second motor neurons: paresis, muscular atrophy fasciculation, emotional lability, spastic paraparesis, tongue muscle atrophy, dysarthria, dysphagia.

frequently. These two phenotypes are characterized by an overall better prognosis, i.e., longer survival. Another special phenotype is progressive bulbar palsy. A distinction between pseudobulbar and bulbar involvement may be difficult, and the leading clinical signs are dysarthria and dysphonia in conjunction with dysphagia, atrophy, fasciculations of the tongue, and sialorrhea (Fig. 1.4). These patients frequently also show pseudobulbar affect. Survival is shorter than that of patients with disease onset in the extremities. Signs of an involvement of the autonomic nerve system, such as reduced perfusion of the extremities, decrease in the heart frequency variability, or changes detected in the electrocardiogram, can be observed. Sensory disturbances and pain are not typical for

ALS, although they have been described. Relevant sensory deficits raise doubts concerning the diagnosis. Respiratory insufficiency develops in the late stages of the disease and is a hallmark of the terminal phase. Loss of body weight frequently occurs early in the disease and may be caused by muscle wasting, dysphagia, and hypermetabolism. Very recently, an association between ALS and frontotemporal dementia has been increasingly discussed. While many patients show mild frontal signs, about 25% may manifest frontotemporal dementia. Depression may develop during the course of the disease and may, at least in some patients, become a relevant clinical aspect. It is not clear whether primary lateral sclerosis (PLS), a disease with selective upper motor neuron signs, is a variant of ALS or a distinct disease. A considerable portion of these patients, however, develop signs of the lower motor neuron over years. Progressive muscular atrophy (PMA) is characterized by pure lower motor neuron signs and otherwise resembles ALS. It has been suggested to regard PMA as a variant of ALS.

## 1.3 The Different Types of ALS

The different types of ALS have different causes. In approximately 5%–10% of patients, the disease is inherited; 20% of these individuals have a mutation of the SOD1 gene, approximately 2%–5% of the TARDBP (TDP-43) gene, and 2%–4% of the FUS/TLS gene. Most patients with ALS, however, have no obvious family history and have sporadic ALS. To date, the only specific marker of sporadic ALS is the presence of inclusions staining positively for ubiquitin and TDP-43 in degenerating motor neurons.

The genetic basis of ALS continues to be investigated (Fig. 1.5). Recently, mutations in the TTP-43 gene have been found to be a cause of some forms of ALS. Mutations in genes often encode proteins that function improperly. Mutations in TTP-43 form proteins that do not properly modify RNA (ribonucleic acid) in motor neurons. This is thought to contribute to the disease process. Identifying the genes and their abnormal protein products helps identify the targets for treatment.

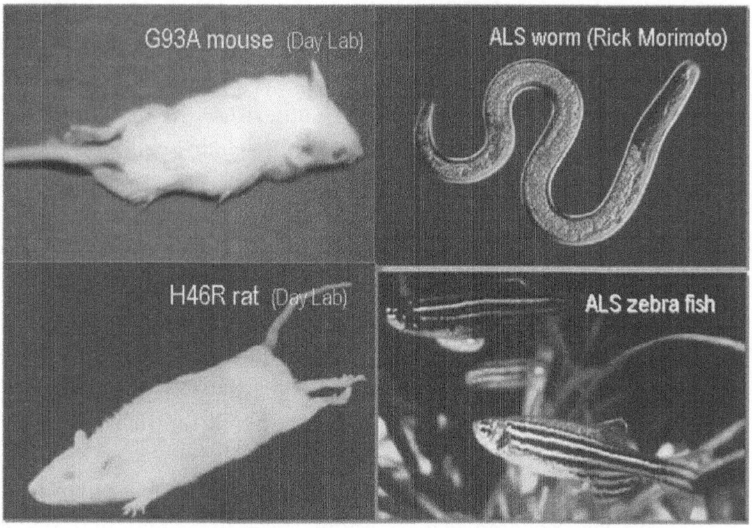


**Figure 1.5** Overexpression of mutant SOD1 generates animal models of ALS. Photos courtesy of Robert Brown, MD, Harvard Medical School, Massachusetts General Hospital. Reprinted with permission.

### 1.3.1 *Familial ALS (Hereditary)*

About 10% of people with ALS have the familial form, which is caused by an inherited genetic mutation. Familial ALS constitutes 5%–10% of all cases of ALS. There are a number of different types of familial ALS, distinguished by genetic cause, age when symptoms begin, and disease progression. They are classified as ALS1-10. Researchers have identified genetic mutations that cause ALS types 1, 2, 4, and 8. Types 1 and 8 are characterized by late-onset symptoms that appear in adulthood. Symptoms of type 1 usually begin between ages 40 and 60 years. Depending on the genetic mutation involved, the condition may progress slowly or rapidly. Symptoms of type 8 ALS begin earlier than type 1 (usually between ages 25 and 44 years) but progress slowly over years to decades. Types 2 and 4 ALS are characterized by early-onset symptoms. Type 2 symptoms usually begin in early childhood or adolescence and slowly worsen over 10 to 15 years. Symptoms of type 4 typically begin before age 25 years and slowly progress over several decades.

Additional types of ALS have been reported, but the mutations that cause them have not been adequately described. ALS1, ALS3, ALS4, ALS6, ALS7, and ALS8 are inherited in an autonomic dominant manner, while ALS2 and ALS5 are inherited in an autosomal recessive manner. Familial ALS with onset in childhood and adolescence (juvenile ALS) is transmitted as an autosomal recessive trait (ALS1:21$q_{22.1}$;ALS3:18$q_{21}$) associated with a mutation of the gene for superoxide dismutase 1 (SOD1), which plays a role in converting cytotoxic oxygen radicals to hydrogen peroxide. It remains unknown how the SOD1 defect causes motor neurons disease. Autosomal dominant inheritance has also been found for ALS plus frontotemporal dementia. ALS together with parkinsonism and dementia occurs among the Chamorro people of Guam.

- ALS1(SOD1). It is caused by mutation in the SOD1 gene on chromosome 21$q_{22.1}$. About 15%–20% of familial ALS is type 1 (ALS1). Linkage analysis in 18 autosomal-dominant; familial ALS pedigrees associated the gene encoding $Cu_{Zn}$ superoxide dismutase (SOD1) on chromosome 21 with ALS. Mutational analysis revealed point mutations in SOD1 to co-segregate with the disease in these pedigrees. The SOD1 protein is a scavenger of free radicals and converts the superoxide anion, a by-product of oxidative phosphorylation in the mitochondrion, to hydrogen peroxide. Interestingly, SOD1 knockout mice do not develop ALS and have a normal life expectancy. It has therefore been hypothesized that mutations lead to a gain of function, perhaps causing mitochondrial dysfunction. However, the mechanism by which SOD1 mutations cause cell death is unknown.

  Mutations in SOD1 have been reported in approximately 12%–23% of familial ALS and 1%–4% of sporadic ALS patients. Subsequent studies have identified over 140 different SOD1 mutations in ALS patients. Most patients with SOD1 mutations have typical ALS, with upper and lower motor neuron involvement, bulbar signs, and a progressive disease course. Patients lacking upper motor neuron signs and with dementia have been reported. Patients with the A4V and D90A substitutions in the protein sequence produce distinctive phenotypes. The A4V mutation is associated with short survival (about 1 year) and limited upper motor neuron involvement.

In northern Scandinavia, the D90A mutation is a benign polymorphism and only individuals homozygous for the mutation develop a form of ALS, characterized by progressive upper motor neuron signs and prolonged survival of more than a decade.

Strikingly, patients with heterozygous D90A mutations outside of Scandinavia develop classic ALS with survival times of 3 to 5 years. It has been hypothesized that a second ameliorating mutation arose on the Scandinavian haplotype, which has not been identified to date.

- ALS2 (ALSin). ALS2 is a juvenile, recessive form of ALS caused by mutation in the gene encoding ALSin on chromosome $2q_{33}$. Linkage analysis in 4 families led to the discovery of an associated locu on chromosome $2q_{33}$ and the identification of the casual mutations in ALSin. Mutations in ALSin have been scarcely reported since its discovery and do not appear to be a common of cause of ALS. Interestingly, mutations in ALSin have also been observed in infantile-onset ascending spastic paralysis and juvenile primary lateral sclerosis.

  The ALSin gene has several guanine-nucleotide exchange factor domains and is a GTPase regulatory protein. These proteins play important roles in signalling pathways, intracellular trafficking, and the organization of the cytoskeleton. Evidence suggests that the identified mutations lead to a loss of function. The phenotype of patients with ALSin mutations is characterized by juvenile onset, hyperreflexia with spasticity of limb and facial muscles, and distal amyotrophy of the hands and feet.
- ALS3 (linkage to locus on 18*q*). This form is an adult-onset ALS due to mutation in a gene on chromosome $18q_{21}$. This locus was identified in a large pedigree with autosomal-dominant, familial ALS, in which 20 individuals were affected. Linkage analysis demonstrated a significant LOD score for a locus on chromosome 18*q* that contains 50

genes. To date, the casual mutation at this locus remains to be identified. All affected individuals presented with a uniform phenotype with disease onset in the legs, disease onset in the midforties, and survival of approximately 5 years. None of the patients showed signs of cognitive impairment.

- ALS4 (SETX). It is a juvenile-onset disease with no bulbar involvement due to mutations in a gene on chromosome $9q_{34}$. This form of familial ALS is a rare, childhood- or adolescent-onset, autosomal dominant disease, which is also known as distal hereditary motor neuronopathy with pyramidal features or dHMN. This locus on chromosome $9q_{34}$ was identified in a large family from Maryland (USA) in which 49 family members were affected. Sequencing revealed a missense mutation in the senataxin gene (SETX) and mutations in this gene could subsequently be identified in additional families with a similar phenotype. SETX has a DNA/RNA helicase domain and has strong homology to genes encoding proteins known to have roles in RNA processing. It is conceivable that the abnormal SETX protein impairs the capacity of neurons to produce error-free mature mRNA, which in turn could lead to neuronal degeneration. It is characterized by low disease progression, limb weakness, severe muscle wasting, pyramidal signs, absence of overt sensory abnormalities, and sparing of bulbar and respiratory muscles.
- ALS5. It is due to mutations in a gene on chromosome 15q15.1-q21.1. ALS5 is the most common form of recessive familial ALS. Linkage to chromosome 15q15-21 was described in seven families from Tunisia and Germany. The locus is a 6 cm segment flanked by microsatellite markers D15S123 and D15S146. To date, the casual mutation at this locus remains to be identified. The phenotype is characterized by atrophy and weakness that initially affects the hands and feet, followed by the tongue and pharynx. Upper motor involvement is moderate in the early stages and becomes more apparent over time.

- ALS6 (FUS). It is due to mutations in a gene on chromosome $16q_{12}$. Linkage to this focus was reported in several kindreds. The associated locus was a 42 Mb region on chromosome 16 containing more than 400 genes. Recently two groups identified mutations in FUS in multiple families that map to this locus. FUS is a predominately nuclear protein that is involved in DNA repair, regulation of transcription, RNA splicing, and export to the cytoplasm. Mutations in FUS lead to cellular mislocalization of the protein and the formation of inclusions, probably resulting in a loss of function.

  Follow-up studies have identified mutations in FUS in familial ALS patients from across Europe and the United States at a frequency of about 5%, making it the second-most prevalent form of familial ALS. The phenotype is characterized by sever signs of lower motor neuron loss and short survival of less than 3 years in most patients.
- ALS7. This form is due to mutations in a gene on chromosome 20p. Linkage to this locus was found in a large, autosomal-dominant, familial ALS pedigree from the United States. In this family, 2 out of 15 siblings were found to be affected and shared a unique 5 Mb segment on chromosome 20p, which contains 24 genes. To date, the mutation at this locus remains to be identified. Patients in this family presented with typical ALS.
- ALS8 (VAPB). This form is due to mutations in a gene on chromosome 20q13.3. The locus is on chromosome 20q13.3. This locus was first identified in a large Caucasian family from Brazil, in which 28 family members were found to be affected across four generations. Sequencing of this region (approximately 1.5 Mb) identified a mutation in the vesicle-associated membrane protein (VAMP)/synaptobrevin-associated membrane protein B gene (VAPB) in all patients of this family. This mutation was subsequently identified in six additional families. A founder effect could be demonstrated and pointed toward a common Portuguese ancestor, indicating that all patients belong to a large genealogy with more than 200 affected

patients and at least 1,300 unaffected relatives. Pathogenic mutations in VAPB have not been reported outside of Brazil. The VAPB protein is thought to play a role in the unfolded protein response, which is an ER housekeeping process that suppresses the accumulation of misfolded proteins. It has been hypothesized that VAPB mutations may cause a decreased unfolded protein response, leading to an accumulation of misfolded proteins in the ER and subsequently cell death.

There are three phenotypes that could be distinguished in patients carrying mutations in VAPB:

- Late-onset SMA. Patients develop limb weakness in the midforties on average and have slow disease progression. The majority of patients were diagnosed 10 years after disease onset. No upper motor neuron signs or bulbar involvement was seen.
- Atypical ALS. Patients presented with a phenotype similar to the late-onset SMA group, but bulbar involvement and upper motor neuron signs were seen as well. Additionally, all patients had an essential tremor.
- Typical ALS. Patients demonstrated upper and lower motor neuron signs with a progressive disease course and survival shorter than 5 years.

  The other forms of ALS are ALS9 (ANG), ALS10 (TARDBP), ALS (DCTN1), ALS-FTD1, ALS-FTD2, which are characterized by angiogenin protein (ANG), TAR DNA-binding protein 43 (TDP-43), chromosome $2P_{13}$, chromosome $9q_{21} - q_{22}$, and $9p_{21.3-13.3}$, with some few cases reported connected to the mitochondrial genes COX1 and IARS2 as well as linkage to the X chromosome, respectively.

In familial ALS, the pattern of inheritance varies with the type. Type 2 ALS is inherited in an autosomal recessive pattern, which means both copies of the gene in each cell have mutations. Most often, the parents of an individual with an autosomal recessive condition each carry one copy of the mutated gene but do not show symptoms of the condition. Types 1, 4, and 8 are inherited in an autosomal dominant pattern, which means one copy of the altered gene in each cell is sufficient to cause the disorder. Studies in Sweden and Finland, however, revealed a small number of type 1 cases that are inherited in an autosomal recessive pattern.

### 1.3.2 *Familial ALS: Signs and Symptoms*

The extra features of familial ALS are eosinophilic intracytoplasmic inclusions in anterior horn cells, degeneration of posterior columns, Clarke's column, and spinocerebellar tracts. Researchers have identified genetic mutations that cause ALS types 1, 2, 4, and 8. Types 1 and 8 are characterized by late-onset symptoms that appear in adulthood. Symptoms of type 1 usually begin between ages 40 and 60 years. Depending on the genetic mutation involved, the condition may progress slowly or rapidly. Symptoms of ALS type 8 begin earlier than type 1 (usually between ages 25 and 44 years) but progress slowly over years to decades. ALS types 2 and 4 are characterized by early-onset symptoms. Type 2 symptoms usually begin in early childhood or adolescence and slowly worsen over 10 to 15 years. Symptoms of type 4 typically begin before age 25 years and slowly progress over several decades. Additional types of ALS have been reported, but the mutations that cause them have not been adequately described.

Each type of familial ALS is caused by mutations in a specific gene. Mutations in the SOD1, ALS2, SETX, and VAPB genes cause ALS type 1, 2, 4, and 8, respectively. How these mutations cause the death of motor neurons and subsequent muscle weakness and atrophy is unclear. Research suggests that these mutations lead to the production of toxic substances or clumps (aggregates) of misshapen proteins that accumulate and damage motor neurons. Another possible explanation is altered development of axons, which are the specialized extensions of nerve cells (such as motor neurons) that transmit nerve impulses. The altered axons may impair transmission of impulses from nerves to muscles. Other genes are thought to contribute to familial ALS, but they have not been identified or fully characterized. For example, mutations in the ANG, DCTN1, NEFH, or PRPH genes, or a reduction in the number of SMN1 or SMN2 genes may also increase the risk of ALS. How variations in these genes contribute to ALS is unclear.

### 1.3.3 *How to Manage Familial ALS?*

Because most ALS is nonfamilial, there is currently little advantage in testing sporadic individual patients for known gene mutations. Genetic testing should only be undertaken in known familial disease, where the presence of mutations in known genes might accelerate the diagnostic process. Genetic counseling is recommended prior to testing. Presymptomatic genetic testing should only be performed in first-degree adult blood-relatives of patients with a known gene mutation. As many mutations in ALS are incompletely penetrant, the identification of a mutation in an asymptomatic relative cannot accurately predict development of the diseases. Testing should be performed on a strictly voluntary basis and should follow extensive genetic counseling.

Good practice points according to the EALSC and EFNS guidelines for diagnosing and good clinical care of ALS patients and relatives:

1. Clinical DNA analysis for gene mutations should only be performed in cases with a known familial history of ALS.
2. Before blood is drawn for DNA analysis, the patient should receive genetic counseling and the time for consideration. DNA analysis should not be performed without the patient's consent.
3. Presymptomatic genetic testing should only be performed in first-degree adult blood-relatives of patients with a known ALS gene mutation.

### 1.3.4 *Sporadic ALS (Acquired)*

Sporadic ALS is a complex disease in which both environmental and genetic factors play a role in the pathogenesis. Most people with ALS have the sporadic form (not inherited). The cause of sporadic ALS is not known, but it probably involves a combination of genetic and environmental factors. Sporadic cases of ALS are sometimes due to new mutation in the SOD1 gene. Despite much effort, the cause of sporadic ALS remains poorly understood, but it probably involves a combination of genetic and environmental factors. Sporadic ALS usually becomes apparent between ages 50 and 70. The presentation is typically with asymmetric weakness of the limbs. Either proximal (difficulty raising the arms or standing up from sitting position) or distal (frequent falls; difficulty grasping, turning a key in a lock) or else with bulbar dysfunction (dysarthria). These deficits are often accompanied by leg cramps and continuous, marked fasciculations in proximal limb muscles. As the disease progresses, weakness, muscular atrophy, dysphgia, and dysarthria become increasingly severe. Respiratory weakness leads to respiratory insufficiency. Spasticity, hyperreflexia, psuedobulbar palsy, emotional liability, and Babinski reflex (inconsistent) are caused by dysfunction of the first motor neuron; muscular atrophy and fasciculations are caused by dysfunction of the second motor neuron; and dysarthria, dysphagia, and weakness are caused by both. The disease progresses rapidly and usually causes death in 3–5 years.

### 1.3.5 *Sporadic ALS: Signs and Symptoms*

The mean age of onset is 60 years, and it begins with impairment of fine finger movement, weakness, and wasting of the muscles of the hand. Later it spreads to the lower limbs, back of the neck, tongue, pharynx, and larynx. The time course is 2–7 years. It is characterized by degeneration of motor neurons in the spinal cord and brainstem and degeneration of pyramidal tracts, loss of Betz cells in some cases, severe atrophy of anterior spinal roots, and intact mental capacity. Neurofilamentous accumulation in cell bodies and proximal axons are a common feature of sporadic and familial cases of ALS.

Despite technical advances in medicine in the last century, the diagnosis of sporadic ALS relies mostly on the interpretation of clinical symptoms and signs (i.e., signs suggestive of combined upper motor neuron and lower motor neuron degeneration, together with disease progression compatible with a neurodegenerative disorder) (Figs. 1.6 and 1.7).

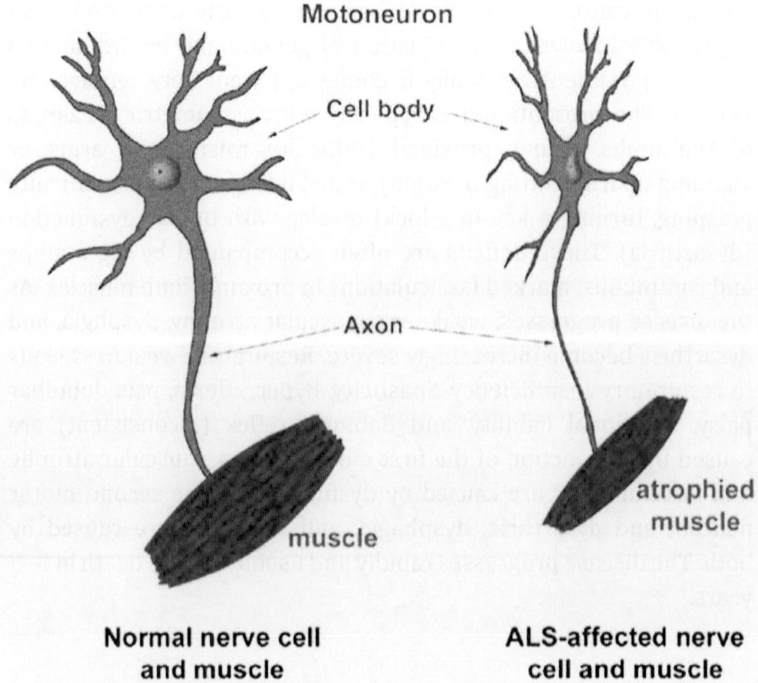


**Figure 1.6** ALS-affected nerve cell with atrophied muscle.

Preclinical and laboratory tests are used only to exclude ALS-mimicking syndromes. In ALS, the absence of a disease marker for UMN and LMN involvement has 2 main negative consequences. First, the delay from onset of the disease to diagnosis of ALS can vary between 13 and 18 months, and the diagnostic delay may even be greater in patients who present with isolated LMN signs. Such a delay precludes early initiation of neuroprotective treatments. Second, the phenotypic heterogeneity of the disease is an important confounding factor in clinical trials (Fig. 1.8).

The cause of sporadic ALS, which makes up 90% of all cases, is not known. The only clear risk factors are age, which is unsurprising given that this is a slowly progressive disease, and having family members with the disease. Because of the latter cause, sporadic ALS may have some genetic basis. In this case, a person with sporadic ALS would have inherited a gene or a pattern of genes that increases

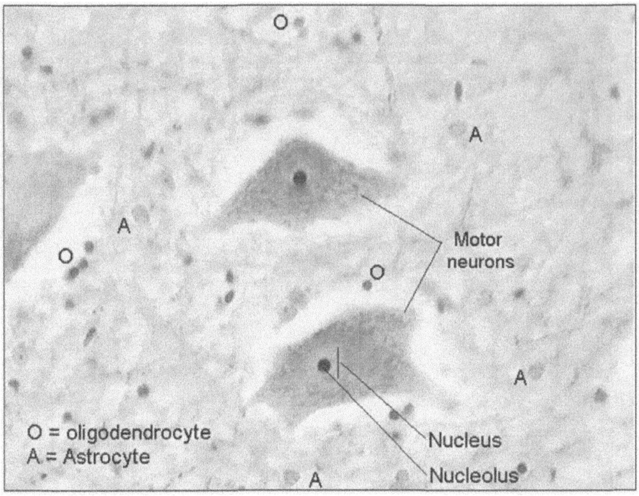


**Figure 1.7** High-power view of motor neurons in MND showing ubiquitinated inclusions. Photograph courtesy of Dr. Martyn Carey. Reprinted with permission.

the risk of developing the disease. The difference between this and familial ALS is that familial ALS is associated with one known gene, which results in a much higher chance of suffering from the disease. The main other possible factors that may increase the risk of developing ALS are cigarette smoking, military service, exposure to lead or other heavy metals, and intensive exercise. These are discussed in Chapter 2 (Fig. 1.9).

In case of ALS variants, the predominant presentation is that seen in sporadic ALS, but includes one or more features such as

1. Familial pattern of inheritance (multiple phenol types characterized by age of onset, site of onset, length of survival, and presumed type of inheritance)

   Familial ALS variants in genetic linkage studies should be characterized by an established genetic mode of inheritance over at least two generations and at least one clinically definite or autopsy confirmed case and compelling evidence excluding other possible causes. Affected subpairs

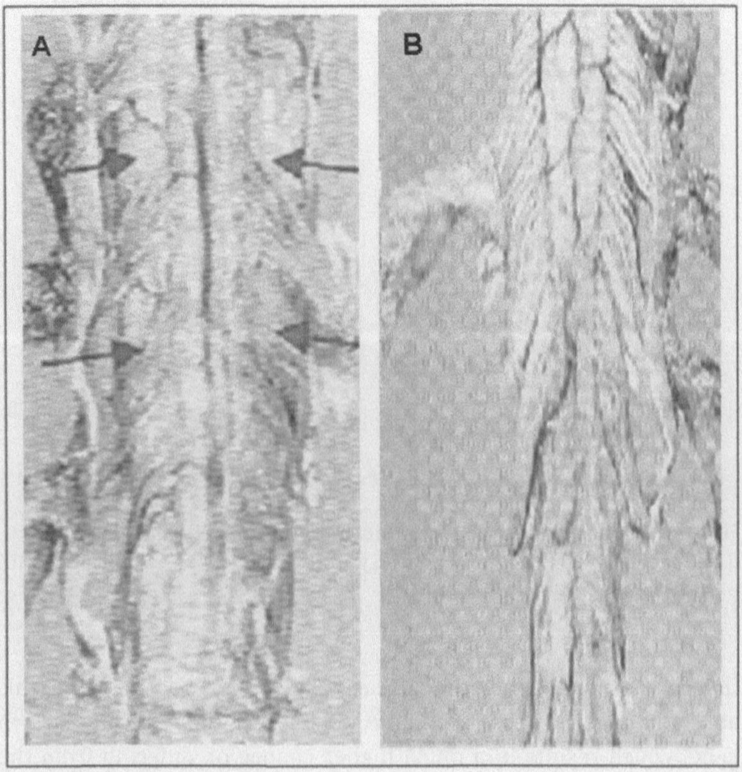


**Figure 1.8** (A) Spinal cord showing loss of motor nerve roots in an ALS patient. The anterior motor nerve roots, indicated by arrows, are severely atrophied. Normal postmortem spinal cord is shown in (B) for comparison. Photograph courtesy of Dr. Marten Carey. Reprinted with permission.

occurring in one generation alone may not result from a single gene effect. Examples:

(a) ALS with defined inheritance and known gene product (hexosaminidase A/B deficiency, superoxide dismutase deficiency)
(b) ALS with defined inheritance and chromosome linkage but no gene product (chromosome 21 associated familial ALS or chromosome 2 associated juvenile familial ALS)

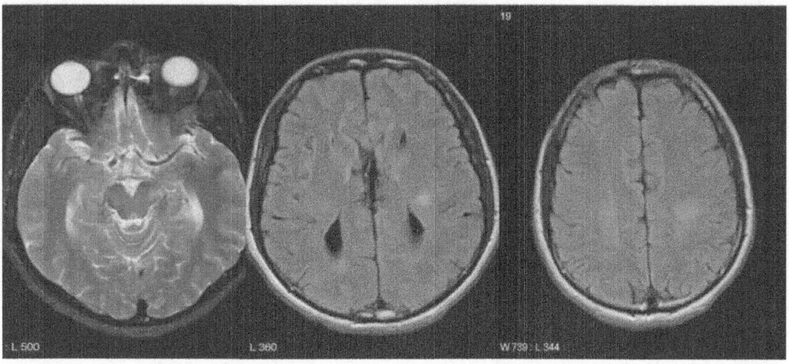

**Figure 1.9** Early unilateral (left) ALS involvement in a patient with associated callosal agenesis.

   (c) ALS with defined inheritance and no known linkage or gene product (most cases or familial ALS)

2. Geographic clustering (including disorders seen in the Western Pacific, Guam, Kii Peninsula, North Africa, Madras, etc.)
3. Extrapyramidal signs (bradykinesia, cogwheel rigidity, tremors, clinically significant onset of supranuclear eye signs [pursuit abnormalities]; familial or sporadic)
4. Cerebellar degeneration (spinocerebellar abnormalities; familial or sporadic)
5. Dementia (progressive cognitive abnormalities; familial or sporadic)
6. Autonomic nervous system involvement (clinically significant abnormal cardiovascular reflexes, bowel or bladder control problems; familial or sporadic)
7. Objective sensory abnormalities (decreased vibration, sharp-dull discrimination, blunting of cold sensation; familial or sporadic)

## 1.4 ALS: Clinical Case Studies

There were 16 families of 20 in which involvement of a parent and her (his) children was reported, 3 families in which involvement of only siblings was reported, and 1 family in which two affected paternal cousins were involved. The sex ratio for the documented familial cases was 0-8:1 (M/F = 12:15), for the total familial (documented + historical) it was 1 (06:1) (33:31), but in sporadic cases it was 1-6:1 (341:212). Familial cases were clinically atypical with a younger mean age of onset (52 years in familial MND; 56 years in sporadic MND) and a shorter median duration of illness (11 years in familial MND; 26 years in sporadic MND). The site of onset of the disease in the two groups was similar: in 44% of sporadic and 48% of familial cases the clinical onset was in an arm; in 37% of each the clinical cases the onset was in a leg. In 19% of sporadic and 15% of familial cases the clinical onset was bulbar. None of these differences, however, reached statistical significance, although, as shown below, they are in agreement with previous reports. There have been frequent reports of preponderance of male to female patients with sporadic MND, with a tendency to the opposite finding in familial cases. Sex ratios of 1-22:25 or more (9:10) for sporadic cases and of 1:1 for familial cases have been reported. A 1:1 ratio has been calculated for sporadic cases older than 65 years. This difference in the sex incidence has not been explained. Both endocrine differences and differences in environmental contacts must be considered.

Past reports also suggest differences in age of onset. In one report, the age of onset was 51 years for familial and 61 years for sporadic cases. In a series of 580 cases the mean age of onset was 52 years for familial and 56 years for sporadic cases. This difference in age of onset might reflect earlier diagnosis of familial MND in patients acquainted with the disease in their parents or siblings. However, the apparently shorter duration in such cases suggests that it is a real phenomenon. The duration of all MND cases from onset to death is usually 3–5 years, although it may be as brief as 1 year or as long as 15 years. From these reported studies the mean survival of familial cases was only −1 year (derived from 22 of 27 cases), while in sporadic cases it was 2–6 years, but unfortunately information was available on only 98 out of 535 cases. It has been suggested that sensory pathways are more often involved in familial cases. This is compatible with the finding that 4 of 20 familial cases had sensory features at presentation, whereas only 5% of sporadic

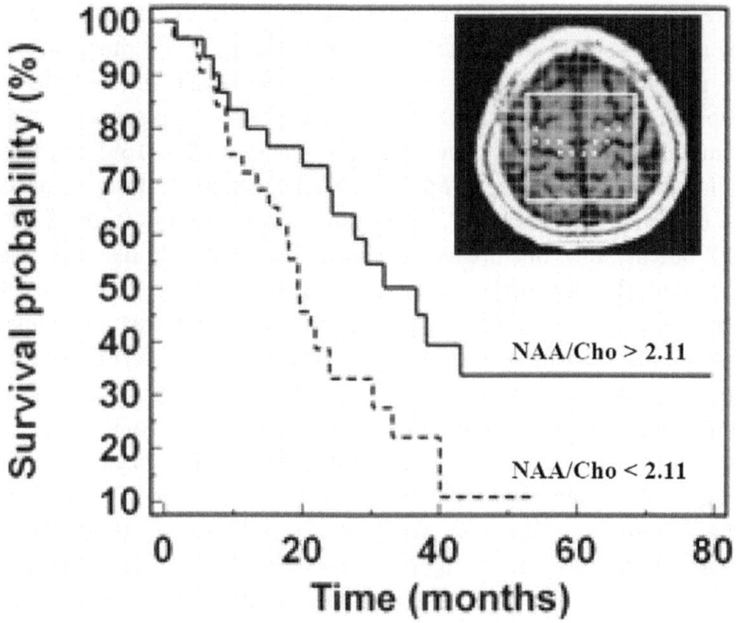


**Figure 1.10** ALS cerebral degeneration predicts survival.

cases had sensory features. Posterior column involvement is well recognized in familial MND. The issue of sensory features in MND is contentious in view of the possibility of a coexisting disorder such as polyneuropathy or cord compression, and since the coexistence of sensory features in a patient thought to have MND is usually held to exclude the diagnosis (Fig. 1.10). The proportion of cases in which the presenting symptoms involved the legs in the present series is consistent with previous studies and was the same in both sporadic and familial MND. In two previous studies, the disease began with weakness in the legs in 40% and 48% of patients with familial MND. In our series the disease presented with weakness of the legs in 37% in both groups. In an earlier study of sporadic MND, 37% (94 out of 255) began in the legs and 28% (72 out of 255) began in the bulbar area.

In a recent study, only 19% of the sporadic cases had a bulbar onset, and the comparable figure for familial cases was 15% pattern of inheritance. A major problem in genetic studies of MND is that the late age of onset of the disease makes it likely that the familial nature of many cases is not ascertained, as many of those theoretically at risk have not reached the usual age of onset at the time of reporting, so that it is likely that the estimate of the proportion of familial cases is always low. In approximately 10%–15% of cases a familial occurrence of MND has been reported. On the basis of documented cases, the proportion in the present study is 5% (27 out of 580), but if cases described in the family histories are included, the proportion increases to 10% (64 out of 617). In 24 families with 124 cases of typical ALS, inheritance was autosomal dominant. According to these studies, the present series parent-to-child transmission occurred in 80%, supporting the theory of autosomal-dominant inheritance. The remaining 20% of these cases probably include genetic disorders possibly inherited in an irregular dominant pattern with incomplete penetrance, but if this were the explanation then one would have to postulate a very low penetrance. However, strong familial clustering, both vertically and horizontally, does not necessarily imply a genetic mechanism. Thus, vertical transmission of an infectious agent, rather than Mendelian inheritance, may explain a familial occurrence of an obscure disease. Furthermore, a genetic analysis of familial MND requires knowledge of metabolic differences between different types of neurons. Such knowledge is very limited at present. For a thorough evaluation of the genetic mechanism, the data would consist, ideally, of the complete family histories of a large group of completely ascertained index cases with a full physical examination collected from a large population. In practice, it is often impossible to ascertain every case in the community, and when retrospective analysis of medical notes is carried out, as in our study, the pedigrees are probably always incomplete, which increases the difficulty of segregation analysis for determining a particular pattern of inheritance. Twin studies 20–23 have not proved helpful.

In summary, although clinical patterns of familial MND overlap with those of sporadic MND, the former appear to be more variable both clinically and, according to the literature, pathologically than sporadic cases. In familial MND the disease may begin at a younger age, and males and females are affected with the same frequency. Although these features indicate that the two groups may differ slightly, the role of familial factors in susceptibility to MND in sporadic cases is unknown and requires further prospective investigation.

## Further Reading


1. Flachenecker P. Epidemiology of neuroimmunological diseases. *J Neurol.* 2006;253(suppl 5):V2–V8.
2. Mayeux R. Epidemiology of neurodegeneration. *Annu Rev Neurosci.* 2003;26:81–104.
3. Liu B, Hong JS. Role of microglia in inflammation-mediated neurodegenerative diseases: mechanisms and strategies for therapeutic intervention. *J Pharmacol Exp Ther.* 2003;304:1–7.
4. Yase Y. The pathogenesis of amyotrophic lateral sclerosis. *Lancet.* 1972;2:292–296.
5. Fang F, Kamel F, Lichtenstein P, et al. Familial aggregation of amyotrophic lateral sclerosis. *Ann Neurol.* 2009;66:94–99.
6. Sreedharan J, Blair IP, Tripathi VB, et al. TDP-43 mutations in familial and sporadic amyotrophic lateral sclerosis. *Science.* 2008; 319(5870):1668–1672.
7. Brugman F, Veldink JH, Franssen H, et al. Differentatiion of hereditary spastic paraparesis from primary lateral sclerosis in sporadic adult-onset upper motor neuron syndromes. *Arch Neurol.* 2009;66:509–514.
8. Pasinelli P, Brown RH. Molecular biology of amyotrophic lateral sclerosis: insights from genetics. *Nat Rev Neurosci.* 2006;7:710–723.
9. Dion PA, Daoud H, Rouleau GA. Genetics of motor neuron disorders: new insights into pathogenic mechanisms. *Nat Rev Genet.* 2009;10:769–782.
10. Ravits JM, La Spada AR. ALS motor phenotype heterogeneity, focality, and spread: deconstructing motor neuron degeneration. *Neurology.* 2009;73:805–811.
11. Greenway MJ, Andersen PM, Russ C, et al. ANG mutations segregate with familial and "sporadic" amyotrophic lateral sclerosis. *Nat Genet.* 2006;38:411–413.
12. Zoccolella S, Beghi E, Palagano G, et al. Predictors of delay in the diagnosis and clinical trial entry of amyotrophic lateral sclerosis patients: a population-based study. *J Neurol Sci.* 2006;250:45–49.

# Chapter 2

# Environmental Factors

Researchers are looking for aspects of lifestyle that can interact with genes to cause or contribute to ALS. The notion that ALS could be linked to viral infection is a concept that reappears periodically when researchers focus on the issue. Exposure to toxins and the influence of intense exertion are ideas researchers consider as possible reasons for the finding that some veterans and some athletes have increased incidence of ALS.

## 2.1 What Environmental Factors Are Suspect in ALS?

After finding the mutated gene for SOD1 in some inherited cases of ALS, researchers continue to search for additional factors that can cause or contribute to the disease. Toxins encountered in the environment have been examined as possible factors in producing the disease. As yet, no conclusive proof exists for any toxin as a causative factor for ALS. Suspects that scientists have researched include heavy metals, solvents, radiation, and electromagnetic fields. As no one would propose to give a known or potentially toxic substance to people on purpose, any study of the potential role of environmental or dietary factors in ALS must be by the methods of

*Amyotrophic Lateral Sclerosis: Advances and Perspectives of Neuronanomedicine*
Lina Machtoub and Yu Kasugai

ISBN 978-981-4463-04-1 (Hardcover), 978-981-4463-05-8 (eBook)
www.panstanford.com

epidemiology. These studies look at populations of people and use answers to questionnaires or information collected from patients and stored in databases to investigate what common factors among people with ALS could provide a link to the disease. Such studies can only reveal a potential association and can never prove cause. Diet and trace minerals in the soil, one of the first clues that ALS might involve an environmental factor, were obtained on the island of Guam in the Pacific, where an unusually high proportion of people over the past century have developed symptoms similar to ALS as they age. Suspects have included trace metals or their lack in the soil, and dietary factors such as the indigenous preference for eating entire bats cooked in coconut milk. No proof has yet nailed down any of these suspects as a cause of ALS. Dietary studies and observations of metal content in tissue from ALS patients do not lend strong support to the role of trace elements, either deficient or excessive in diet (Figs. 2.1 and 2.2).

| ***Factor*** | ***Odds Ratio*** |
|---|---|
| ***Toxins*** | |
| *Agricultural Toxins* | |
| -- herbicides | 3.0 |
| -- fertilizers | 2.3 |
| *Metals* | |
| **-- lead exposure** | **1.6** |
| *Respiratory* | |
| -- smoking | 3.3 |
| *Infectious Agents* | |
| **-- retroviruses** | |
| -- Lyme | |
| **-- other** | |
| *Diet* | |
| -- high fat | 3.8 |
| -- high glutamate | 3.2 |
| **-- high fiber** | **0.3** |
| Exercise | 2-6 |

**Figure 2.1** The development of ALS reflects an interplay of environmental, genetic, and aging factors.

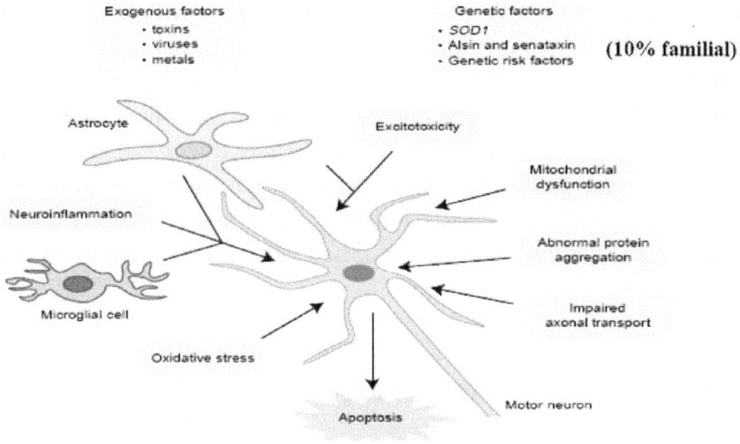


**Figure 2.2** Schematic diagram of the pathophysiological mechanisms of ALS.

## 2.2 Toxic Metals and Solvents

Many investigations of heavy metal exposure, particularly lead, and including mercury and manganese, have looked at risk factors for ALS. A positive association between past exposure to heavy metals and risk of ALS has not consistently appeared across studies. These studies include occupational exposure that epidemiologists often use as a surrogate to assess potentially toxic exposures. Many of the studies relied on self-reporting by questionnaires. Self-reports can allow a recall bias—I have this disease, what did I do to produce it—that has the potential to artificially inflate the data. Some support for an association between ALS and exposure to organic solvents appears in epidemiological studies, yet these have found only weak association and a mix of positive and negative results. As well, no consistent associations with ALS have emerged from investigation into the potential role of radiation and electromagnetic fields.

Besides the Chamorro people of Guam, U.S. veterans are another group of people who appear to develop ALS more often than the general population. A study found that the relative risk of dying from ALS for veterans was 1.5 times than seen for men who did not serve. The increased risk was apparent for veterans of World War II, the

Korean War, and the War in Vietnam. A prior study had found that the rate of ALS in young Gulf War veterans was more than two times greater than expected for the general population. Scientists have expressed concern that the degree of excess risk is not convincing because of the small number of total ALS cases documented in these studies of veterans. Statistical theory says that such small numbers may not be able to provide reliable answers to questions about associations between diseases and their causes. Larger sample sizes are needed for better certainty.

## 2.3 The Possible Effects of Exercise or Pesticides

One idea that researchers offer is that soldiers on active duty are engaged in strenuous physical labor. Or, they are exposed to toxins which could play a role in ALS. The ALS Association is helping to fund an effort by the Veterans Administration (VA) to collect information about veterans diagnosed with ALS, to shed light on possible environmental factors associated with the disease. This VA registry will also serve as a stepping stone to clinical trials. Both possibilities, of toxin exposure or the influence of intense exertion, are advanced when researchers consider the finding that Italian soccer players appear to have increased incidence of ALS. It remains unclear whether exercise is indeed a risk factor and what types of exercise may be of concern. Indeed some studies seem to suggest that a degree of exertion may be beneficial in ALS. Other ideas are that pesticides or some other chemical encountered on maintained playing fields might be involved.

## 2.4 Environmental Influences of Viruses

A recurring idea about environmental influences on ALS is that a virus is responsible for the condition. Polio virus, for instance, infects motor neurons and can at times lead to a weakening condition called the post-polio syndrome years after the initial infection. Scientists have considered viral infection for many other disorders of the nervous system, from schizophrenia to multiple sclerosis, as well as for ALS. A concrete link to viral infection has never been documented in any of these diseases.

The ALS Association has recognized the debate over a viral role in ALS and has funded study of the issue, but so far findings have failed to confirm any link with ALS and viral infection. The Association will continue to support investigations into the way that environmental factors may interact with genetics to produce ALS.

## 2.5 BMAA Neurotoxic Effects

BMAA (methylamino-L-alanine) is considered a possible cause of the amyotrophic lateral sclerosis/parkinsonism dementia complex (ALS/PDC), which has an extremely high rate of incidence among the Chamorro people of Guam. The Chamorro call the condition lytico-bodig. In the 1950s, ALS/PDC prevalence ratios and death rates for Chamorro residents of Guam and Rota were 50 to 100 times that of developed countries, including the United States. No demonstrable heritable or viral factors were found for the disease, and a subsequent decline of ALS/PDC after 1955 on Guam led to the search for responsible environmental agents. The use of cycad (Cycas circinalis) seeds in food and traditional medicine had decreased as the Chamorro population became more Americanized following World War II. In addition to direct consumption in the form of seeds, BMAA may have found its way into human diet by way of biomagnification. Fruit bats, a Chamorro delicacy, may feed on cycad seeds and concentrate the toxin in their flesh. Three museum specimen bats, collected in Guam in the 1950s, contained hundreds of times more BMAA, gram for gram, than cycad seeds. Recent studies have begun to shed light on the effects of BMAA and the possible link to ALS and Alzheimer's.

In 2009 neuroscientist from the University of Miami (UM) conducted an independent study of ALS and Alzheimer's brains using samples from the brain bank. The results that followed were shocking: BMAA was found in 23 out of the 24 samples derived from 12 Alzheimer's patients, and all 13 samples that were taken from ALS patients tested positive for BMAA. Studies like this one are still being conducted to see if the results can be reproduced to show that there is a link between BMAA and ALS and Alzheimer's. Unequivocal evidence implicating BMAA as a causative factor in human sporadic or familial ALS and AD has not been forthcoming. The multifocal nature of neurodegenerative processes in human ALS and AD suggests multiple etiologies.

In recent studies high concentrations of BMAA have been discovered in shark fin, a neurotoxin possibly linked to neurodegenerative diseases in humans, including Alzheimer's and Lou Gehrig's disease (ALS). The study suggests that consumption of shark fin soup and cartilage pills may pose a health risk for degenerative brain diseases, but further research is necessary.

Degenerative locomotor diseases had been described in animals grazing on cycad species, fueling interest in a possible link between the plant and the etiology of ALS/PDC. Subsequent laboratory investigations discovered the presence of BMAA, which induced severe neurotoxicity in rhesus macaques, including limb muscle atrophy nonreactive degeneration of anterior horn cells, degeneration and partial loss of pyramidal neurons of the motor cortex, behavioral dysfunction, conduction deficits in the central motor pathway, and neuropathological changes of motor cortex Betz cells. There are reports that low BMAA concentrations can selectively kill cultured motor neurons from mouse spinal cords. In the motor neurons, BMAA activates AMPA-kainate glutamate receptors and boosts production of oxygen radicals.

The presence of BMAA in cyanobacteria, among the most populous organisms in the world, has raised concerns that humans worldwide may be exposed to levels of BMAA that could be potentially harmful. Cyanobacteria from soil and water samples collected around the world produce BMAA, giving rise to speculative biomagnification in food chains. Scientists have also found that newborn rats treated with BMAA show early neurotoxicity and impaired learning and memory as adults.

## 2.6 Are Toxins in Seafood Causing ALS?

What started as the discovery of an unknown disease in Guam has spread to a line of ominous findings about some of our most debilitating conditions and potential toxins lurking in bodies of water around the world. There have been several studies to understand that risk by tracking how BMAA moves through the food chain in Florida waters where regular cyanobacteria blooms occur. It has been shown that only few of the fish and shellfish specimens contain BMAA. Bottom feeders registered notably high, perhaps because cyanobacteria accumulate not only on the ocean surface but also along the seafloor. Compared with the amount of BMAA found in the fruit bats of Guam, the levels of the toxin Brand found in Florida oysters and mussels were moderate. But pink shrimp, largemouth bass, and blue crabs—all eaten by humans—contained levels comparable to or even exceeding those in the bats. One blue crab topped the charts with 7000 parts per million of BMAA, twice as much toxin as found in a Guam bat, but blue crabs collected from bloom areas in the Chesapeake Bay had similarly high levels of BMAA. In recent studies, Swedish researchers also found the neurotoxin in bottom-feeding fish living in the Baltic Sea, a hotbed for cyanobacteria blooms, although at lower levels than seen in the Chesapeake Bay and along the Florida coast. The correlations between BMAA and neurological disease seem strong, but as skeptics point out, correlation does not prove causation. And that is just one problem they have with Cox's theory.

The field has been dogged by clashing findings, leading some critics to question whether BMAA truly is a potent neurotoxin. Furthermore, there is no known mechanism that can explain how an amino acid that is alien to human biology could travel across the blood–brain barrier, get incorporated into proteins, and then trickle out to cause disease.

It has been recently reported that even if BMAA may increase the risk, it appears unlikely to be a major factor behind neurological disorders like ALS and Alzheimer's. Most experts think these brain afflictions have multiple causes, including genes, poor diet, lack of exercise, and a variety of environmental agents, including pathogens and pesticides. It has been indicated that the overall risk from BMAA is probably low and only a few people are genetically at risk, and that even if BMAA causes common disorders like Alzheimer's and Parkinson's, that still doesn't mean we should shun seafood. Commercial fishermen generally do not work in areas heavily contaminated with cyanobacteria, so the danger of exposure in the United States and Canada should be modest for those who eat typical store-bought or homegrown food and avoid drinking contaminated water.

Recent studies have been carried on ALS clusters on the Kii Peninsula in southeastern Japan. The data suggest that ALS is 2.5 times more common than average within one-half mile of a lake or pond where cyanobacteria have bloomed. It has been hypothesized that people living around the lakes may have breathed in BMAA from the air, eaten fish contaminated with it, or accidentally swallowed it while swimming. Test were conducted of brain bank tissue to see if the ALS patients in these regions do in fact have elevated levels of BMAA. While the evidence mounts, researchers are already thinking about ways to detect toxic exposure before it causes disease. Reports recall the intriguing case of a woman who died of an ALS-like illness called progressive supranuclear palsy. For decades before her death, she had a habit of cutting her hair, dating it, and putting it in her diary. Since virtually everything consumed leaves a trace residue in hair, as an opportunity to see if the woman had been exposed to BMAA, her hair was examined and it was discovered that the hair had been accumulating the toxin as early as 1939, with the level creeping upward over the next two decades. By 1957 the neurotoxin had reached the kind of abundance that is measured in Alzheimer's patients. The amount peaked around 1962 and then began to decrease, with none detectable at the time of the woman's death.

In this context ALS is generally viewed as distinct clinicopathological entities. Outside specific geographical regions such as the island of Guam and the Kii Peninsula of Japan, the combination of ALS and Parkinson's disease is highly unusual. Furthermore, western Pacific parkinsonism-dementia complex/ALS (PDC-ALS) is pathologically distinct from common Parkinson's disease and ALS because of the abundance of Alzheimer-type neurofibrillary tangles. In the Western world, the rare cases of ALS with nigral degeneration that have been reported are referred to as ALS-plus. Combinations of neurodegenerative disorders reported include progressive supranuclear palsy (PSP) and Parkinson's disease, PSP and multiple system atrophy (MSA), ALS and the cerebellar form of MSA, and the combination of Alzheimer's disease, Parkinson's disease, ALS, and diffuse Lewy bodies in a single patient. Bearing in mind that many such cases go unreported, it is tempting to believe that the co-occurrence of multiple neurodegenerative disorders is more frequent than would be expected by chance. Some cases have been reported of patients who presented with clinical features of both Parkinson's disease and amyotrophy. At necropsy, the patients were found to have the hallmark pathological features of three distinct neurodegenerative disorders marked by tau, $\alpha$-synuclein, and ubiquitin inclusions. The clinical and pathological features along with the common underlying mechanisms of inclusion formation and protein aggregation are still under investigation.

The incidence of ALS is approximately 2 per 100,000 population per year in most Western countries, although there are a few isolated areas in the world, such as Guam (USA), the Kii Peninsula (Japan), and Irian Jaya (Indonesia), in which ALS is more prevalent. Males appear to be affected more than frequently than females, with a ratio of 1.6:1.0. The average age of onset is in late fifties, but ranges from 18 to well over 80 years of age.

In the Kii Peninsula (Japan), Muro disease is an endemic ALS in the Muro district that includes the southern coastal mountainous areas of the Kii Peninsula. Epidemiological survey in 1960s disclosed extremely high incidence of ALS in two villages, Hohara and Kozagawa, and disappearance of high incidence by early 1980s was reported with its etiology unsolved. It has been found that ALS and parkinsonism-dementia complex (PDC) frequently occurred in one individual simultaneously and affected many members in the same family. The neuropathological findings of ALS and PDC were similar to each other, showing a combination of upper and lower motor neuron involvement and many neurofibrillar tangles in the brain stem and cerebral cortex, resembling those of ALS/PDC in Guam.

Age-adjusted incidence rates during 1950 and 2000 have showed that incidence of ALS was gradually declining for 50 years. Continuing high incidence and high rates of familial occurrence suggest that the primary cause of Kii ALS/PDC may be genetic rather than environmental.

## Further Reading


1. Kimura K. Studies of amyotrophic lateral sclerosis in the Kozagawa district of the Kii peninsula, Japan. *Wakayama Med Rep* 1965;9:177–192.
2. Kurland LT, Mulder DW. Epidemiologic investigations of amyotrophic lateral sclerosis. I. Preliminary report on geographic distribution, with special reference to the Mariana Islands, including clinical and pathologic observations. *Neurology* 1954;4:355–378.
3. Kithara T, Yoshida S, Hironishi M, Miwa H, Okamato K, Kondo T. Changes in the incidence of amyotrophic lateral sclerosis in Wakayama, Japan. *Amyotroph Lateral Scler Other Motor Neuron Disord.* 2005;6:155–163.
4. Logroscino G. Incidence of amyotrophic lateral sclerosis in Europe. *J Neurol Neurosurg Psychiatry* 2010;81:385–390.
5. World Fedration of Neurology Subcommittee on Motor Neuron Disease. El Escorial World Fedration of Neurology criteria for the diagnosis of amyotrophic lateral sclerosis. *J Neurol Sci* 1994;124(suppl):98–107.
6. Saito Y, Yokota T, Mitani T, et al. Transgenic small interfering RNA halts amyotrophic lateral sclerosis in a mouse model. *J Biol Chem* 2005;280:42826–42830.
7. Wolfson C, Kilborn S, Oskoui M, Genge A. Incidence of amyotrophic lateral sclerosis in Canada. *Neuroepidemiology* 2009;33:79–88.
8. Chio A, Mora G, Calvo A, et al. Epidemiology of ALS in Italy: a 10-year prospective population-based study. *Neurology* 2009;24:725–731.
9. Nishimura AL, Mitne-Neto M, Silva HC, et al. A mutation in the vesicle-trafficking protein VAPB causes late-onset spinal muscular atrophy and amyotrophic lateral sclerosis. *Am J Hum Genet* 2004;75:822–831.
10. Ravits JM, La Spada AR. ALS motor phenotype heterogeneity, focality, and spread: deconstructing motor neuron degeneration. *Neurology* 2009;73:805–811.
11. Millul A, Beghi E, Logroscino G, et al. Survival of patients with amyotrophic lateral sclerosis in a population-based registry. *Neuroepidemiology* 2005;25:114–119.

# Chapter 3

# Diagnostic Criteria of Amyotrophic Lateral Sclerosis

The diagnosis of ALS relies on the simultaneous presence of signs and symptoms of damage of the upper and lower motor neurons, which in most patients are rapidly progressive and lead to death by respiratory failure within two to four years. Other classical diagnostic features are the focal onset of the diseases which progressively spread to the entire voluntary motor system and the presence of fasciculations. The latter aspect of the disease leads to a false positive diagnosis of ALS if benign fasciculations are misinterpreted as unequivocal signs of the disease. In clinical practice, the diagnosis of ALS can be made using medical history, physical examination, and diagnostic tests.

## 3.1 Steps in the Diagnosis of ALS

ALS cannot be detected by a blood test. Laboratory tests are used to eliminate other possible diagnoses. For this reason, muscle enzyme creatine kinase (CK) is tested to make sure the weakness is not due to muscle disease. Blood tests also rule out organ failure, cancer, and upset of the body chemistry (metabolic disturbance)

*Amyotrophic Lateral Sclerosis: Advances and Perspectives of Neuronanomedicine*
Lina Machtoub and Yu Kasugai

ISBN 978-981-4463-04-1 (Hardcover), 978-981-4463-05-8 (eBook)
www.panstanford.com

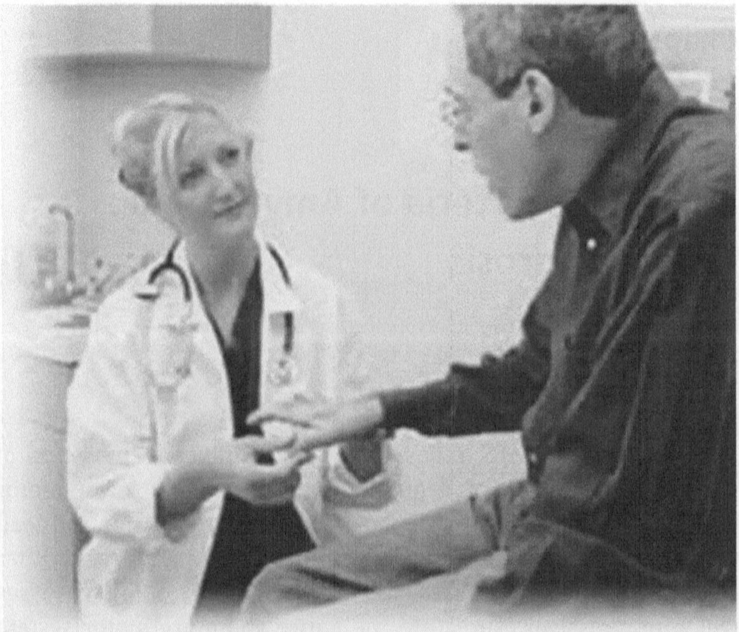

**Figure 3.1** Tests. Healthcare providers would run thorough neurological examination to diagnose ALS based on electrodiagnostic tests, including electromyography and nerve conduction velocity, blood and urine studies, spinal tap, x-rays, and muscle and/or nerve biopsy.

(Fig. 3.1). The diagnosis of ALS is made possible by following history, physical, and appropriate neurological examinations to ascertain clinical findings, which may suggest suspected, possible, probable, or definite ALS; electrophysiological examinations to ascertain findings which confirm LMN degeneration in clinically involved regions, identify LMN degeneration in clinically uninvolved regions, and exclude other disorders; neuroimaging examinations to ascertain findings which may exclude other disease processes; clinical laboratory examinations, determined by clinical judgment, to ascertain possible ALS-related syndromes; neuropathological examinations, where appropriate, to ascertain findings which may confirm or exclude sporadic ALS, coexistent sporadic ALS, ALS-related syndromes, or ALS variants; and repetition of clinical and electrophysiological examinations at least six months apart to ascertain evidence of progression.

### 3.1.1 *History and Physical Exam*

Progressive weakness in the large central muscles, like the pectoral muscles and buttock muscles, as well as in the small, distant muscles of the fingers and toes is suggestive of ALS. However, ALS does not cause unusual sensations, numbness, or tingling, and it does not cause pain. If these symptoms are present, another condition is most likely present.

Physical examination helps doctors assess the symptoms, especially weak, shrunken, or twitching muscles. These symptoms are caused by a loss of motor neurons that connect to muscles, the lower motor neurons. Reflexes are often increased because of the loss of upper motor neurons (motor neurons in the brain). The diagnosis of ALS depends on finding evidence that both upper and lower motor neurons are affected.

### 3.1.2 *Electrophysiology Studies*

Electrophysiology studies the electrical impulses from the brain, nerves, and muscles. It studies how well the nerves and body conduction systems work. It involves placing stimulators on the scalp, peripheral nerves, and muscles and measuring the waveform of the signals that are conducted away. In ALS the conduction between the brain, nerves, and muscles is reduced in many different muscles. These studies can be used to estimate the number of nerve cells and fibers in each nerve. The number is always reduced in ALS.

In the absence of an established biological marker, ALS is primarily a clinical diagnosis. In patients with generally increased reflexes, weak and wasted muscles in several body regions, a progressive history, often after a focal onset, the diagnosis is readily established after appropriate imaging and other tests designed to exclude other possible diagnoses. An experienced clinician may be virtually certain of the diagnosis in a patient with bilateral limb wasting, bilateral fasciculation in the tongue, or wasting and hyperreflexia limited to a single limb, but none of these syndromes meets established criteria for a definite diagnosis of ALS.

Clinical neurophysiological examination is especially important in this context, because it can extend the clinical findings by revealing lower motor neuron involvement in muscles in body regions, otherwise regarded as unaffected. An algorithm for utilizing electrophysiological data in diagnosis was incorporated in the revised El Escorial criteria for the diagnosis of ALS as laboratory-supported ALS. However, as currently understood, EMG and clinical abnormalities cannot be combined in a single limb. Rather, the limb must be determined to be abnormal by one technique or the other. Another factor that has limited the utility of clinical neurophysiology in the diagnosis of ALS is that current criteria require that muscles determined to be affected must show both ongoing denervation, defined by fibrillation potentials (fibs) or positive sharp waves (sw), and chronic partial reinnervation, implying reinnervation, defined by enlarged, frequently unstable motor units of increased duration, with a reduced interference pattern. While the presence of active denervation and chronic denervation/reinnervation in the same muscle, although not specific for ALS, is diagnostically useful, many muscles do not show fibs-sw, so that the clinical neurophysiologist is left with insufficient findings to make the diagnosis of ALS. In practice this is a significant problem; on current criteria, 22% of patients with ALS may die without reaching a level of diagnosis more certain than possible ALS. It has become increasingly important to diagnose ALS early in the natural history of the disease in order to arrange best management. It is intuitively likely that disease-modifying agents will be most successful when administered early, when a large population of motor neurons remains viable. Although specific disease-modifying therapy is presently of limited efficacy, symptomatic treatments provide considerable benefit. In addition, the pace of translational research in ALS promises an increasing number of experimental therapies, with opportunities to enter clinical trials.

Up to now the diagnosis ALS is still a clinical one, and EMG is the most important technical test to support the diagnosis. Laboratory tests and imaging, including MRI, do not yield diagnostically positive results, but are necessary to exclude other potentially better treatable diseases.

The gold standard of ALS diagnosis are the El Escorial criteria (EEC) as revised in 1998. These criteria are mainly based on clinical findings, although they appreciate results of electrophysiological studies. The EEC are, however, fairly rigid and allow a diagnosis only relatively late in advanced stages of the disease. This has been criticized particularly by experts active in treatment trials of ALS as it appears reasonable to include patients in earlier stages of the disease, when the EEC do not yet allow a diagnosis. For this reason, several experts in the field of ALS and of electromyography suggested a new set of diagnostic criteria, the so-called Awaji criteria, which are based on the El Escorial criteria, but modify some of their statements to EMG findings and therefore increase the diagnostic sensitivity (Figs. 3.2 and 3.3).

## *The El Escorial Criteria initiated by the WFN*

In order to standardize the diagnosis of ALS, the El Escorial Criteria (EEC) were developed in 1994 following the older Airlie House criteria. The EEC were revised in 1998. They are mainly clinical and form the gold standard of ALS diagnosis. They are, however, relatively rigid and are not suitable for early diagnosis. They are important for scientific classification and, so far, for recruitment into clinical trials, but not for clinical praxis. According to the EEC, the diagnosis of ALS requires the presence of A criteria and the absence of B criteria:

---

1. For the evaluation of LMN disease in ALS in any given body region clinical and electrophysiological abnormalities have equal diagnostic significance
2. EMG features of chronic neurogenic change must be found, for example
   (a) MUPs of increased amplitude and increased duration, usually with an increased number of phases, as assessed by qualitative or quantitative studies
   (b) Decreased motor unit recruitment, defined by rapid firing of a reduced number of motor units. In limbs affected by clinical features of significant UMN abnormalities, rapid firing may not be achieved
   (c) Using a narrow band pass filter (500 Hz to 5 kHz) unstable and complex MUPs will be observed in most cases of ALS
3. In ALS fbs-sw are usually recorded in strong, non-wasted, muscles
4. In the presence of chronic neurogenic change on needle EMG in ALS, fasciculation potentials (FPs), preferably of complex morphology, are equivalent to fibrillations and positive sharp waves (fibs-sw) in their clinical significance

---

**Figure 3.2** Criteria for detection of neurogenic change by needle EMG in the diagnosis of ALS. Reproduced with permission from Carvalho et al., *Clinical Neurophysiology* 119 (2008), 497–503.

1. Principles (from the Airlie House criteria)

The diagnosis of amyotrophic lateral sclerosis [ALS] requires

*(A) the presence of*

(1) evidence of *lower motor neuron (LMN) degeneration* by clinical, electrophysiological or neuropathological examination

(2) evidence of *upper motor neuron (UMN) degeneration* by clinical examination; *and*

(3) *progressive spread of symptoms or signs* within a region or to other regions, as determined by history, physical examination, or electrophysiological tests

*(B) the absence of*

(1) *electrophysiological or pathological evidence of other disease processes* that might explain the signs of LMN and/or UMN degeneration, and

(2) *neuroimaging evidence of other disease processes* that might explain the observed clinical and electrophysiological signs

2. Diagnostic categories

*Clinically definite ALS* is defined by *clinical or electrophysiological* evidence by the presence of LMN as well as UMN signs in the bulbar region and at least two spinal regions or the presence of LMN and UMN signs in three spinal regions

*Clinically probable ALS* is defined on *clinical or electrophysiological* evidence by LMN and UMN signs in at least two regions with some UMN signs necessarily rostral to (above) the LMN signs

*Clinically possible ALS* is defined when *clinical or electrophysiological* signs of UMN and LMN dysfunction are found in only one region; or UMN signs are found alone in two or more regions; or LMN signs are found rostral to UMN signs. Neuroimaging and clinical laboratory studies will have been performed and other diagnoses must have been excluded

These recommendations emphasize the equivalence of clinical and electrophysiological tests in establishing neurogenic change in bodily regions. The category of "Clinically Probable Laboratory-Supported ALS" is rendered redundant.

**Figure 3.3** Awaji-shima consensus recommendations for the application of electrophysiological tests to the diagnosis of ALS, as applied to the revised El Escorial Criteria (Airlie House, 1998). Reproduced with permission from Carvalho et al., *Clinical Neurophysiology* 119 (2008), 497–503.

## A criteria

A1: Degeneration of the lower motor neuron approved by clinical, electrophysiological, or neuropathological examination

A2: Degeneration of the upper motor neuron approved by clinical examination

A3: Progressive dissemination beyond typical nerve supply areas

## B criteria

B1: Electrophysiological or neuropathological findings typical for other diseases which could explain the degeneration of the upper and lower motor neurons

B2: Findings in imaging studies which can explain the clinical symptoms

The diagnosis of ALS requires an extensive history and a thorough clinical and electrophysiological examination. The electrophysiological tests can demonstrate the involvement of the lower motor neurons in affected and frequently also in clinically unaffected body regions. The EEC define four body regions to be evaluated:

- bulbar (brain stem)
- cervical (neck and upper extremities)

- thoracal (trunk and abdominal wall)
- lumbosacral (lumbar spine and lower extremities)

### 3.1.3 *Radiology Studies*

Radiology studies include x-rays and scans. The most important radiology study in ALS is the magnetic resonance imaging (MRI) scan of the brain and spine. MRI takes very high resolution pictures of the inside of the brain and the spinal cord, which contains high numbers of upper motor neurons. The main use of MRI is to rule out other conditions that can mimic, or appear very similar to, ALS. These include compression of the spinal cord from a slipped disc or fracture of the spine, as well as strokes and multiple sclerosis. Unlike with these other conditions, an MRI scan appears normal in a person with ALS.

#### Conventional MR imaging findings

Routine anatomic imaging of the brain and/or the spinal cord is helpful in ruling out diseases that mimic ALS with varying degrees of UMN and LMN signs. The revised criteria of the World Federation of Neurology Research Group on Motor Neuron Diseases state that conventional MR imaging studies are not required in cases that have a clinically definite disease with a bulbar or a pseudobulbar onset. On the other hand, in patients with clinically probable or possible ALS, MR imaging can be useful in excluding several ALS mimic syndromes, including cerebral lesions (e.g., multiple sclerosis and cerebrovascular disease), skull base lesions, cervical spondylotic myelopathy, other myelopathies (e.g., foramen magnum lesions, intrinsic and extrinsic tumors, and syringomyelia), conus lesions, and thoracolumbar sacral radiculopathy.

In patients with ALS, signal intensity changes on conventional MR imaging (i.e., T2-weighted, PD-weighted, and FLAIR sequences) can be observed along the corticospinal tract (CST). Typically, CST changes, which are best followed on coronal scans, appear as areas of bilateral increased signal intensity from the centrum semiovale to the brain stem. However, the frequency of CST hyperintensities in patients with ALS varies significantly in different studies (ranging

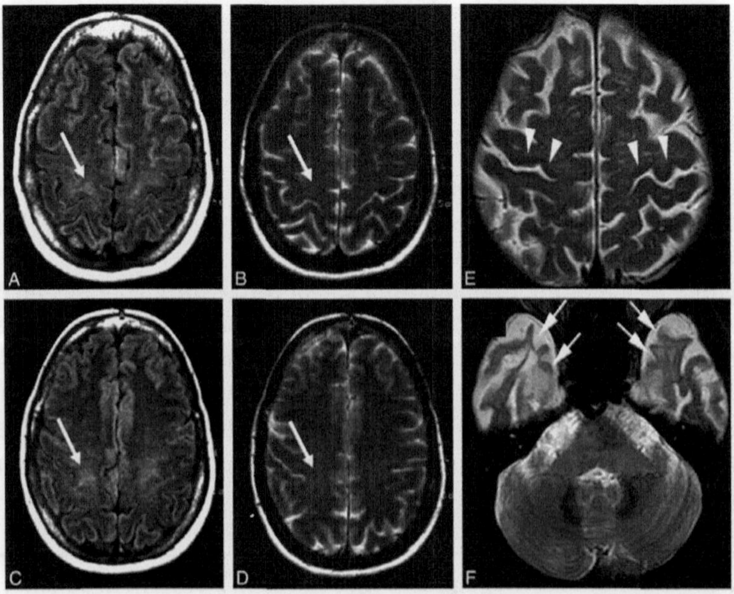


**Figure 3.4** Conventional MR imaging findings in patients with ALS. A–D: Hyperintensity at the subcortical precentral gyrus (A and B) and the centrum semiovale (C and D) on FLAIR (arrows A and C) and T2-weighted (arrows B and D) images of a 66-year-old patient with ALS. Modified with permission from Hecht et al. E and F: T2-weighted images obtained from a 58-year-old patient with ALS with dementia show hypointensity along the precentral cortices (arrowhead E) and symmetric hyperintensity in the anterior temporal subcortical WM (arrow F). A and D reproduced with permission from the *Journal of the Neurological Sciences* (2001), 186:37–44. Copyright 2001, Elsevier Ltd.

from 15% to 76%), and it is not yet clear which may be the most sensitive MR image to detect them (Fig. 3.4). The combined application of T2-weighted, PD-weighted, and FLAIR images has recently reached a sensitivity of approximately 62%. In addition, CST signal-intensity changes do not correlate with clinical scores. More remarkably, CST hyperintensities have also been described in healthy subjects, and in patients with other conditions, such as Krabbe disease, X-linked Charcot–Marie–Tooth neuropathies, and adrenomyeloneuropathy. In patients with ALS, a characteristic low signal intensity (hypointense rim) of the precentral cortex on T2-

weighted images can be observed. However, such a change is neither sensitive nor specific to the pathology of ALS.

Symmetric T2 signal-intensity changes in the anterior temporal subcortical white matter have been described in patients with ALS and dementia. Pathologically, such hyperintensities correspond to loss of myelin, white matter degeneration, and gliosis. Significant lower whole brain volume has been found in patients with ALS relative to healthy controls. Global brain atrophy is, however, relatively mild. Consistent with pathologic data, T2 and T1 hyperintensities of the anterolateral columns of the cervical cord have been observed in patients with ALS. Such hyperintensities are likely to have higher specificity than signal-intensity changes on brain MR images. T1 hyperintensity of the anterolateral cervical cord has been associated with a younger age and a rapid disease progression.

### Nonconventional MR imaging assessment of motor system regional atrophy

Despite the consistent finding of cortical motor involvement in pathologic studies of ALS, in vivo MR imaging studies did not reach firm conclusions regarding the presence of motor/premotor cortical atrophy (Fig. 3.5). Using voxel-based morphometry (VBM) to assess the regional distribution of white matter loss, researchers have found atrophy of the corticospinal tract (CST) in patients with ALS, which was more severe in patients with a bulbar onset. Patients with ALS showed atrophy of the cervical cord relative to controls, which significantly worsened during a 9-month follow-up.

### 1H-MR spectroscopy

In patients with ALS, 1H-MR spectroscopy studies demonstrated a decrease in NAA (*N*-acetylaspartate) concentrations. The physiologic role of NAA in the central nervous system remains unclear. However, because NAA appears to be present only in neurons of the adult human brain and in their processes, the content of NAA is used as a biochemical marker of neuronal integrity. These findings have been recently confirmed at 3T. However, the diagnostic value of 1H-MR spectroscopy is poor because of the considerable overlap of the metrics of patients with those of healthy controls.

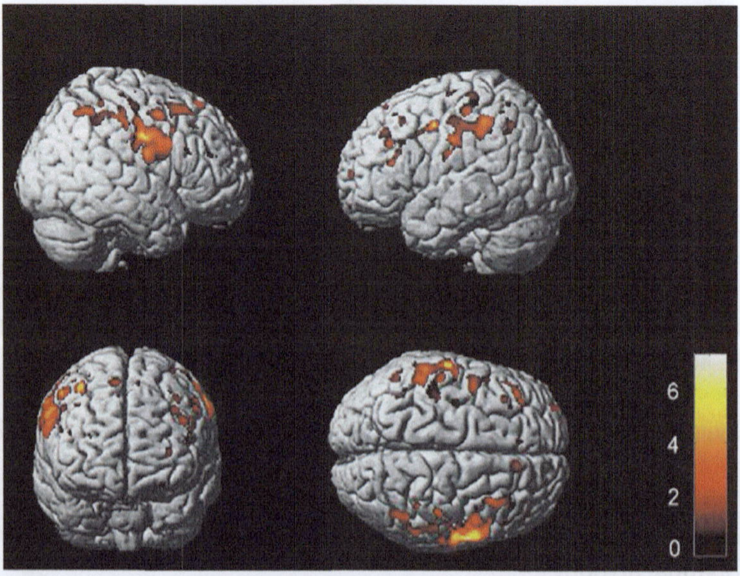


**Figure 3.5** Regional gray matter (GM) atrophy in patients with ALS compared with controls. A group comparison of 17 patients with ALS versus 17 healthy controls shows regional GM atrophy in the precentral and postcentral gyri bilaterally, which extends from the primary motor cortex to the premotor, parietal, and frontal regions bilaterally (displayed at $P = 0.001$, uncorrected; extended threshold, 100 voxels). The color bar represents the $t$-score. The differences between groups are superimposed on a standard normalized T1-weighted image. Images are shown in neurologic convention.

Patients with ALS showed decreased NAA/Cr and NAA/Cho ratios along the CST. Although the regional analysis of these data showed more pronounced 1H-MR spectroscopy changes in the precentral gyrus and corona radiata, NAA reduction in the brain stem has also been reported. Cross-sectional studies have shown a moderate correlation between NAA concentration (and its ratios) in the motor cortex cortex and clinical manifestations of ALS (i.e., disease severity, extent of UMN signs, and maximum finger tapping rate). Patients with bulbar onset have the most severe pattern of motor cortex 1H-MR spectroscopy changes compared with those with a limb onset. In addition to neuronal damage, increased glial cell activity, reflected by raised levels of myo-inositol (mIns), has been demonstrated in the motor cortex of patients with ALS. Increased mIns levels are associated with motor cortex hypointensity on T2-weighted images. In a 3T 1H-MR spectroscopy study of patients with ALS, the NAA/mIns ratio provided better sensitivity and specificity for detecting disease than the individual metabolites and was the strongest correlation with disease severity.

Using either region of interest-based approaches or tractography, DTI studies of patients with ALS reported consistently decreased FA and increased MD values along the CST. Loss of pyramidal motor neurons in the primary motor cortex and axonal degeneration of the CST, together with the proliferation of glial cells, extracellular matrix expansion, and intraneuron abnormalities, may contribute to the observed CST DTI changes. The most pronounced decreased FA and increased MD have been shown in the posterior limb of the internal capsule. Decreased FA in patients with ALS was found to correlate with disease severity, rate of disease progression, and clinical and electrophysiologic measures of UMN involvement. Patients with a bulbar onset exhibited the most marked FA decrease. In two studies, increased MD of the CST was associated with disease duration. Compared with controls, patients with ALS had significantly lower FA of the cervical cord, which was strongly associated with the ALSFRS scores. This finding indicates the presence of distortion of cord tissue geometry in ALS and agrees with pathologic data showing a pronounced cord degeneration and a reduction in the number of LMNs in the anterior horns of the cord GM in patients with ALS.

During motor tasks, fMRI demonstrated an increased activation of the contralateral sensorimotor cortex and the supplementary motor area. Increased sensorimotor activation was also reported in the hemisphere ipsilateral to the movement. A spatial shift of recruitment to more anterior regions of the premotor cortex during upper limb movement was also observed in patients with ALS (Fig. 3.6). In patients with ALS, increased activation of the inferior parietal cortex during a motor task has been reported. A relationship with task difficulty or a compensatory role of these motor-related areas has been suggested.

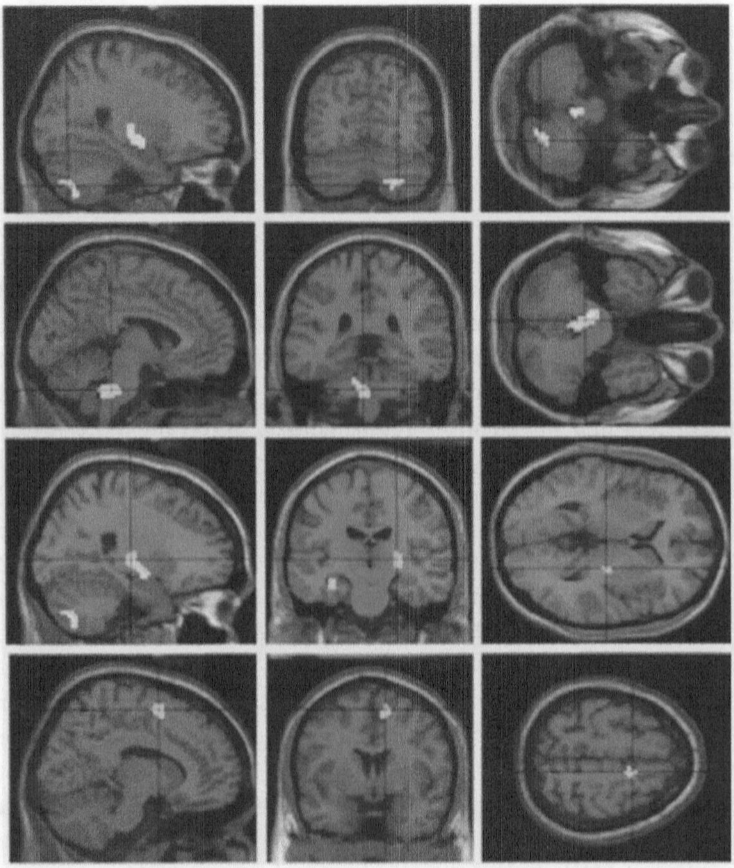

**Figure 3.6** Brain regions showing a significant increased recruitment on fMRI scans from 10 patients with ALS relative to 10 healthy controls during right-handed movement ($P < 0.05$, small volume correction). Modified with permission from Konrad et al., *Experimental Brain Research* (2006), 172:361–369. Copyright 2006, Springer Science.

The motor execution in ALS has been also associated with increased activations of areas involved in motor learning, such as the basal ganglia and the cerebellum. It is suggested that an increase in movement-associated cortical activations beyond the primary motor cortex is associated with the degree of UMN involvement.

## 3.2 Electrophysiology in the Revised EEC

The revised EEC state that EMG/NCV (nerve conduction velocity) examination is an extension of the clinical examination used to identify LMN dysfunction, which can be defined by electromyographic concentric needle examination to provide evidence of active and chronic denervation. Signs of active denervation consist of fibrillation potentials and positive sharp waves, while fasciculation potentials are not mentioned in this context. Signs of chronic denervation consist of large motor unit potentials of increased duration with an increased proportion of polyphasic potentials often of increased amplitude and reduced interference pattern with firing rates higher than 10 Hz, unless there is a significant UMN component, in which case the firing rate may be lower than 10 Hz and the motor unit potentials unstable. The EEC also state that the combination of active denervation findings and chronic denervation findings is required but that the relative proportion may vary from muscle to muscle. Fasciculation potentials are mentioned in the revised EEC as a characteristic clinical feature of ALS, but are not used for clinical or electromyographical diagnosis. Their presence in EMG is considered helpful in the diagnosis of ALS, especially if they reveal a neurogenic configuration (long duration and polyphasicity) and when they are present in muscles in which there is evidence of active or chronic partial denervation and reinnervation.

## 3.3 Nerve Conduction Studies

The EEC point out that nerve conduction studies are required in the diagnosis of ALS to exclude motor neuropathy or other disorders of peripheral nerves, the neuromuscular junction, and muscles that may mimic or confound the diagnosis of ALS. In this context it is worthwhile to mention that an especially difficult differential diagnosis can be multifocal motor neuropathy (MMN) with conduction blocks. The EEC state that motor conduction times should be normal, unless the compound muscle potential is small. Sensory nerve conduction studies should be normal although they can be changed in the presence of entrapment syndromes and other coexisting peripheral nerve disease. In addition, lower extremity sensory nerve responses can be abnormal in the elderly.

## 3.4 Clinical Features in the Diagnosis of ALS

Patients with signs of LMN degeneration (weakness, atrophy, and clinical fasciculations) and UMN degeneration (spasticity, pathologic reflexes, etc.) may be suspected as having ALS. Careful history as well as physical and neurological examination must search for further clinical evidence of LMN and UMN signs in four regions of the central nervous system.

1. Signs of LMN degeneration (weakness, wasting, and fasciculations) in one or more of the four regions (bulbar, cervical, thoracic, and lumbosacral). LMN findings in a region are without regard to right or left, but those for another region are more important than spread from right to left or vice versa.
2. Signs of UMN degeneration (increased or donic tendon reflexes, spasticity, pseudobulbar features, Hoffmann reflex, and extensor plantar response) in one or more of the four regions. These UMN signs are clinically best appreciated in the bulbar, cervical, and lumbosacral regions. UMN findings in a region are also without regard to right or left. Once the physical and neurological examinations provide information on the presence or absence of LMN and UMN signs in the four regions (bulbar, cervical, thoracic, and lumbosacral), they must be ordered topographically so as to determine the certainty of the diagnosis of ALS.
3. The topographical location of certain UMN and LMN signs in the four regions of the CNS. This determines the certainty of the diagnoses of ALS. Progression is a cardinal feature of the clinical diagnosis of ALS. Progression of signs within a region and progression of signs to involve other regions are crucial to the diagnosis.

   Clinical examinations should be repeated at least every six months to assess progression.

> Cases which meet the topographical criteria for probable or definite ALS but which lack progression during the 12-month period diagnosis should be designated as possible ALS.

Definite ALS is defined on clinical grounds alone by the presence of UMN as well as LMN signs in the bulbar region and at least two of the other spinal regions or the presence of UMN and LMN signs in three spinal regions. An important determinant of the diagnosis of definite ALS in the absence of electrophysiological, neuroimaging, and laboratory examinations is the presence of UMN and LMN signs together in multiple regions.

Probable ALS is defined on clinical grounds alone by UMN and LMN signs in at least two regions. While these regions may be different, some UMN signs must be rostral to (above) the LMN signs. Multiple combinations of UMN and LMN signs may be present in patients with probable ALS.

Possible ALS is defined on clinical grounds alone when the UMN and LMN signs are in only one region or UMN signs alone are present in two or more regions or LMN signs are rostral to UMN signs (the latter distribution of signs needs to be differentiated from multiple non-ALS processes).

Monomelic ALS, progressive bulbar palsy without spinal UMN and/or LMN signs, and progressive primary lateral sclerosis without spinal LMN signs constitute special cases which may develop LMN or UMN signs to meet the criteria for probable ALS with time or be subsequently confirmed at autopsy by specific LMN and UMN neuropathologic findings.

Suspected ALS will manifest only LMN signs in two or more regions, although UMN pathology might be demonstrated at autopsy. However, only clinical signs are considered pertinent to this classification at the time of diagnostic evaluation.

The clinical features that support the diagnosis of ALS include one or more of the following:

1. abnormal pulmonary function test not explained by other causes
2. abnormal speech studies not explained by other causes
3. abnormal swallowing studies not explained by other causes

4. abnormal larynx function studies not explained by other causes
5. abnormal isokinetic or isometric strength test in clinically uninvolved muscles
6. abnormal muscle biopsy with evidence of denervation

## 3.5 Inconsistent Clinical Features

Clinical findings inconsistent with the diagnoses of ALS include one or more of the following not explained by physiological changes associated with aging or other disease processes:

1. sensory dysfunction
2. sphincter abnormalities
3. autonomic nervous system dysfunction
4. anterior visual pathway abnormalities
5. movement abnormalities associated with probable Parkinson's disease defined by DATATOP criteria
6. cognitive abnormalities associated with clinical Alzheimer's disease as defined by NINCDS-ADRDA criteria

If these clinical findings occur, then close attention should be paid to the possible diagnosis of other disease processes. LMN and UMN signs may occur together with other clinical signs in disease where the pathologic process is not primary motor neuron degeneration.

The physical and neurological examinations will allow for the clinical diagnosis of ALS to a particular degree of certainty as defined above. However, the history of the disease onset, toxic exposures, past medical history, injuries, family history, geographic location, etc., must be incorporated with the clinical examinations in determining whether the patient may have an ALS-related syndrome or an ALS variant.

ALS-related syndromes must meet the clinical, electrophysiological, and neuroimaging criteria for possible, probable, or definite ALS. ALS-related syndromes have unique laboratory-defined or epidemiologically defined features which are time-linked to the development of the ALS phenotype. If correction of the associated laboratory-defined feature does not result in correction of the ALS phenotype, then the patient with an ALS-related syndrome should be considered in the same way as a patient with sporadic ALS.

ALS-related syndromes include

1. monoclonal gammopathy (monoclonal gammopathy of unknown significance, Waldenstrom's macroglobulinemia, osteosclerotic myeloma, etc.)
2. dysimmune motor system degeneration (autoimmune, high-titer GMI ganglioside antibody, etc.)
3. nonmalignant endocrine abnormalities (hyperthyroidism, hyperparathyroidism, hypogonadism, etc.)
4. lymphoma (Hodgkin's and non-Hodgkin's lymphoma). Cases of sporadic ALS associated with insulinoma, lung, colon or thyroid cancer are thought not to be casually related
5. Infection (HIV-1, HTLV-I, encephalitis lethargica, varicella-zoster, brucellosis, cat-scratch disease, Creutzfeldt–Jakob disease, syphilis, delayed post-poliomyelitis, etc.)
6. acquired enzyme defects (detoxification enzymes, etc.)
7. exogenous toxins (lead, mercury, arsenic, thallium, cadmium, manganese, aluminum, organic pesticides, lupin seeds, etc.)
8. physical injury (electric shock, radiation therapy, etc.)
9. vasculitis (ischemic) (Dejerine anterior bulbar artery syndrome, etc.)
10. spondylotic myelopathy (painless myelopathy with no sensory signs, stabilization or progression post surgery)

ALS variants must meet the clinical, electrophysiological, and neuroimaging criteria for possible, probable, or definite ALS.

## 3.6 ALS Electrophysiological Features

Patients with suspected, possible, probable, or definite ALS on clinical grounds should have electrophysiological studies performed to confirm LMN degeneration in clinically affected regions, to find electrophysiological evidence of LMN degeneration in clinically uninvolved regions, and to exclude other pathophysiological processes. ALS may be most reliably identified when the clinical and electrophysiological findings are widespread, involving a sufficient number of regions, so that other possible causes of similar EMG abnormalities are highly unlikely. The confirmation of the diagnosis of ALS depends on finding electrophysiological evidence of LMN degeneration in at least two muscles of different root or spinal nerves and cranial or peripheral nerve innervation in two or more of the four (bulbar, cervical, thoracic, and lumbosacral) regions. The features of LMN degeneration in a particular muscle are defined by electromyographic needle examination and nerve conduction studies using standard methods for each measure. Electrophysiological features required to identify definite primary LMN degeneration include all of the following:

1. reduced recruitment (reduced interference pattern with firing rates over 10 Hz)
2. large motor unit action potentials (large amplitude, long duration) (Fig. 3.7)
3. fibrillation potentials

Electrophysiological features that support the identification of possible primary LMN degeneration include one or more of the following:

1. either reduced recruitment, large motor unit potentials, fibrillation potentials or unstable motor unit potentials alone
2. polyphasic motor unit potentials or increased single fiber density alone
3. low-amplitude compound muscle action potentials if the disease duration is over 5 years or if there is associated atrophy
4. compound muscle action potential change between proximal and distal sites of stimulation that is uniform along the length of the nerve
5. up to 30% decrement in motor conduction velocity below established normal values if a low-amplitude compound muscle action potential greater than 10% of normal is present
6. up to 50% decrement in motor conduction velocity below established normal values if the compound muscle action potential is below 10% or normal

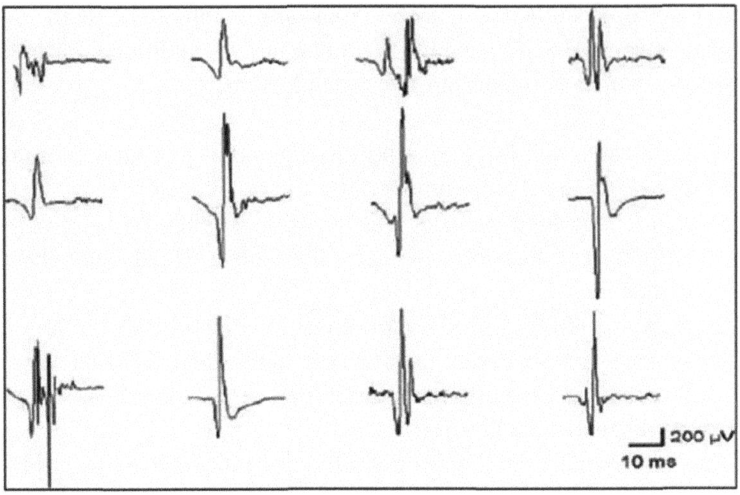


**Figure 3.7** Motor unit action potentials obtained from the bicep muscle of a patient with early ALS at slight innervation. Amplitudes are frequently higher than 1 mV and the configuration is frequently polyphasic.

7. up to 20% decrement of the compound muscle action potential on 2 Hz repetitive stimulation
8. up to 10% decrement in sensory nerve conduction velocity and action potential amplitude from established normal values
9. complex repetitive discharges
10. absence of fasciculations

Electrophysiological features compatible with UMN degeneration and not excluding ALS include one or more of the following:

1. up to 30% increment in central motor conduction velocity
2. up to 10% decrement in somatosensory, evoked potential amplitude, and up to 10% increment in somatosensory-evoked potential latency
3. mild abnormalities of autonomic function
4. mild abnormalities of polysomnography
5. mild abnormalities of electronystagmography

Electrophysiological features that are inconsistent with the diagnosis of ALS or suggest the presence of additional disease processes include one or more of the following:

1. focal reduction in compound muscle action potential or more than 10% in a 4 cm segment
2. motor conduction velocities, F-wave latencies, or H-wave amplitudes which are more than 30% above established normal values
3. more than 20% decrement of repetitive stimulation at 2 Hz
4. sensory action potential latencies more than 20% above or sensory action potential amplitudes more than 20% below established normal values
5. unstable motor unit potentials with no other electromyographic changes
6. more than 30% increment of central motor conduction velocity
7. more than 10% increment in sensory-evoked potential latency or more than 10% decrement in sensory-evoked potential amplitude
8. moderate or greater abnormalities in autonomic function or electronystagnography

Employing electrophysiological evidence of LMN degeneration to confirm the diagnosis of ALS

The certainty of LMN degeneration is determined by the presence of the above findings for each muscle tested in the region. At least two muscles of different root or spinal nerve and different cranial or peripheral nerve inneveration in each region should show electrophysiological evidence of either definite, probable, or possible LMN degeneration for that region to be ranked as showing definite, probable, or possible.

The definite LMN degeneration by EMG has the same significance as clinical LMN degeneration and can upgrade the certainty of the clinical diagnoses of ALS in the same fashion as if the clinical signs of LMN degeneration were present in that region. Probable or possible LMN degeneration by EMG does not carry the same weight as either clinical signs or definite electrophysiological evidence of LMN degeneration in a particular region. However, the involvement of the regions with probable electrophysiological evidence of LMN degeneration or one region with probable and one region with possible electrophysiological evidence of LMN degeneration carries the same weight as one region with definite evidence of LMN degeneration in upgrading the certainty of diagnosis of ALS.

A single region with electrophysiological evidence of probable LMN degeneration or two regions with electrophysiological evidence of possible LMN degeneration can be used to upgrade the certainty of the diagnosis of ALS from possible ALS to probable ALS, but not from probable ALS to definite ALS.

## 3.7 ALS Neuroimaging Features

Neuroimaging studies should be selected in order to exclude other conditions which may cause UMN and/or LMN signs that may stimulate sporadic ALS.

Neuroimaging features required for the diagnosis of ALS: there are no neuroimaging tests which confirm the diagnosis of ALS. Neuroimaging features that support the diagnosis of ALS include one or more of the following:

1. minimal bony abnormalities on plain x-ray of the skull or spinal canal
2. minimal abnormalities on head or spinal cord MRI scans without spinal cord and/or root compression
3. minimal abnormalities on spinal cord myelography with post-myelography CT tomography showing no spinal cord and/or root compression

Neuroimaging features that are inconsistent with the diagnosis of ALS include one or more of the following:

1. significant bony abnormalities on plain x-ray of the skull or spinal canal
2. minimal abnormalities on head or spinal cord MRI scans without spinal cord and/or root compression

3. minimal abnormalities on spinal cord myelography with post-myelography CT tomography showing no spinal cord and/or room compression

Somre more neuroimaging features that are inconsistent with the diagnosis of ALS include one or more of the following:

1. significant bony abnormalities on plain x-rays of skull or spinal canal that might explain clinical findings
2. significant abnormalities of head or spinal cord MRI suggesting intraparenchymal processes, arteriovenous malformations, or compression of the brainstem or spinal cord and/or cranial nerve or spinal nerve roots by bony abnormalities, tumor, etc. MRI of craniocervical function if bulbar onset and/or MRI of pertinent spinal region if spinal onset
3. significant abnormalities of spinal cord myelography with or without CT tomography or CT tomography alone suggesting lesions as noted above
4. significant abnormalities on spinal cord angiography suggesting arteriovenous malformations

The absence of abnormalities in appropriately performed neuroimaging studies will raise the possibility of patients with clinical and/or electrophysiological evidence of probable ALS to being diagnosed with definite ALS. On the other hand, the absence of neuroimaging abnormalities cannot increase the chance of possible ALS to probable ALS.

In summary, the extensive application of modern neuroimaging techniques to the study of ALS has undoubtedly improved our understanding of disease pathophysiology and may have a role in the identification of potential biomarkers of disease progression. Nevertheless, there are many remaining challenges. New techniques need to be harnessed and integrated into clinical research and practice. New acquisition schemes and analysis procedures require standardization and optimization so that they can be used in multiple settings, both in natural history studies and treatment trials. From recent studies, it is evident that combining different imaging modalities that are sensitive to different aspects of ALS pathology (e.g., motor and extramotor) is a promising way to further increase our understanding of the mechanisms accounting for the accumulation of irreversible disability in this condition.

## Further Reading


1. Tucker K, Robertson KR, Lin W, et al. Neuroimaging in human immunodeficiency virus infection. *J Neuroimmunol* 2004;157:153–162.
2. Dhib-Jalbut S, Arnold DL, Cleveland DW, et al. Neurodegeneration and neuroprotection in multiple sclerosis and other neurodegenerative diseases. *J Neuroimmunol* 2006;176:198–215.
3. Kuwabara Y. Advance of SPECT: differential diagnosis and evaluation of pathophysiology of neurodegenerative disorders. *Rinsho Shinkeigaku* 2004;44:894–896.
4. Silverman DH, Alavi A. PET imaging in the assessment of normal and impaired cognitive function. *Radiol Clin North Am* 2005;43:67–77.
5. Wearne SL, Rodriguez A, Ehlenberger DB, Rocher AB, Henderson SC, Hof PR. New techniques for imaging, digitization and analysis of three-dimensional neural morphology on multiple scales. *Neuroscience* 2005;136:661–680.
6. Kantarci K, Smith GE, Ivnik RJ, et al. 1H magnetic resonance spectroscopy, cognitive function, and apolipoprotein E genotype in normal aging, mild cognitive impairment and Alzheimer's disease. *J Int Neuropsychol Soc* 2002;8:934–942.
7. Burn DJ, O'Brien JT. Use of functional imaging in Parkinsonism and dementia. *Mov Disord* 2003;18(suppl 6):S88–S95.
8. Thurnher MM, Castillo M, Stadler A, Rieger A, Schmid B, Sundgren PC. Diffusion-tensor MR imaging of the brain in human immunodeficiency viruspositive patients. *AJNR Am J Neuroradiol* 2005;26:2275–2281.
9. Walker Z, Walker RW. Imaging in neurodegenerative disorders: recent studies. *Curr Opin Psychiatry* 2005;18:640–646.
10. Block W, Träber F, Flacke S, Jessen F, Pohl C, Schild H. In-vivo proton MR-spectroscopy of the human brain: assessment of N-acetylaspartate (NAA) reduction as a marker for neurodegeneration. *Amino Acids* 2002;23:317–323.
11. Bhanu Prakash K, Gupta V, Bilello M, Beauchamp NJ, Nowinski WL. Identification, segmentation, and image property study of acute infarcts in diffusion-weighted images by using a probabilistic neural network and adaptive Gaussian mixture model. *Acad Radiol* 2006;13:1474–1484.

12. Goodin DS, Rowley HA, Olney RK. Magnetic resonance imaging in amyotrophic lateral sclerosis. *Ann Neurol* 1988;23:418–420.
13. Lule D, Ludolph AC, Kassubek JM. I-based functional neuroimaging in ALS: an update. *Amyotroph Lateral Scler* 2009;10:258–268.
14. Andersen PM, Borasio GD, Dengler R, et al. EFNS task force on management of amyotrophic lateral sclerosis: guidelines for diagnosing and clinical care of patients and relatives. *Eur J Neurol* 2005;12:921–938.
15. Hecht MJ, Fellner F, Fellner C, et al. Hyperintense and hypointense MRI signals of the precentral gyrus and corticospinal tract in ALS: a follow-up examination including FLAIR images. *J Neurol Sci* 2002;199:59–65.
16. Agosta F, Chio A, Cosottini M, et al. The present and the future of neuroimaging in amyotrophic lateral sclerosis. *AJNR Am J Neuroradiol* 2010;31:1769–1777.
17. Kassubek J, Unrath A, Huppertz HJ, et al. Global brain atrophy and corticospinal tract alterations in ALS, as investigated by voxel-based morphometry of 3-D MRI. *Amyotroph Lateral Scler Other Motor Neuron Disord* 2005;6:213–220.
18. Mezzapesa DM, Ceccarelli A, Dicuonzo F, et al. Whole-brain and regional brain atrophy in amyotrophic lateral sclerosis. *AJNR Am J Neuroradiol* 2007;28:255–259.

# Chapter 4

# Perspectives of Neuronanomedicine

Medical nanotechnology has made broad incremental contributions to improving the effectiveness of existing drugs, diagnostics, prosthetics, patient monitoring, and personal health care maintenance. The evolutionary growth of nanomedicine arose from research that progressed from the micro- to the nanoscale, and from the molecular scale back up to the nanoscale. Now, nanoparticle-based therapeutics is poised to have significant impact on the treatment of neurodegenerative diseases. In this chapter, we aim to attract interdisciplinary attention for future integration of the recent nano-based biotechnological achievements with the clinical need of early diagnosis and complete cure for neurodegenerative diseases.

## 4.1 Nanomedicine and Neurological Disorders

The recently growing application of nanotechnology in molecular detection of biomarkers is promising for very early diagnosis of neurodegenerative diseases. From a practical point of view, it has become possible to perform a molecular detection process either inside the body (in vivo) or on the samples derived from the body (in vitro). Nanotechnology is suggesting approaches to improve the

*Amyotrophic Lateral Sclerosis: Advances and Perspectives of Neuronanomedicine*
Lina Machtoub and Yu Kasugai

ISBN 978-981-4463-04-1 (Hardcover), 978-981-4463-05-8 (eBook)
www.panstanford.com

sensitivity of both in vitro and in vivo molecular detections for neurological disorders. This application of nanotechnology in molecular diagnosis is mainly due to the special physical, chemical, and biological characteristics of nanoparticles for signal transduction. Signal transduction refers to the process through which a biological signal (a biomarker) transforms to a recordable signal. This process usually includes some degree of signal amplification. The controllable properties (optical, electrical, magnetic, or biological) of certain nanostructures make them suitable for the transformation and amplification of biological signals. In this section, we aim to discuss the latest research studies on neuronanomedicine and nanodiagnostic approaches for neurodegerative diseases in terms of special applications.

En route to very early diagnosis of a complex disease like ALS, we need to have an affordable, ultrasensitive, and selective molecular detection method. Nanotechnology may help us to achieve this by providing us with a highly potent molecular amplification and signal transformation through in vitro and/or in vivo methods. In what follows, we present and compare a number of methods that have aimed to address this need. Pathological conditions affecting the brain such as neurodegenerative diseases and neurological disorders are among the most untreatable syndromes. A great number of pharmacologically active molecules are not able to reach the CNS to exert their pharmacological activity as they cannot cross the BBB (Fig. 4.1). As widely described in the past, the blood–brain barrier (BBB) was thought of as a static barrier, permeable only to lipophilic or small hydrophilic molecules. Nowadays, the BBB is correctly described as a very dynamic interface, with several transport systems (influx systems), able to trigger the BBB crossing of a variety of molecules circulating in the bloodstream (hydrophilic and lipophilic, with high or low molecular weights). The influx systems could also trigger the passage of macromolecules by exploiting endocytosis or transcytosis mediated by specific receptor interactions. Along with these influx systems, at the BBB level, efflux systems are present, protecting the brain from damaging agents and xenobiotic exposure, thus defending the brain from toxic insults. Unfortunately, it is estimated that approximately 98% of drugs active against brain pathologies do not cross the BBB. As a consequence,

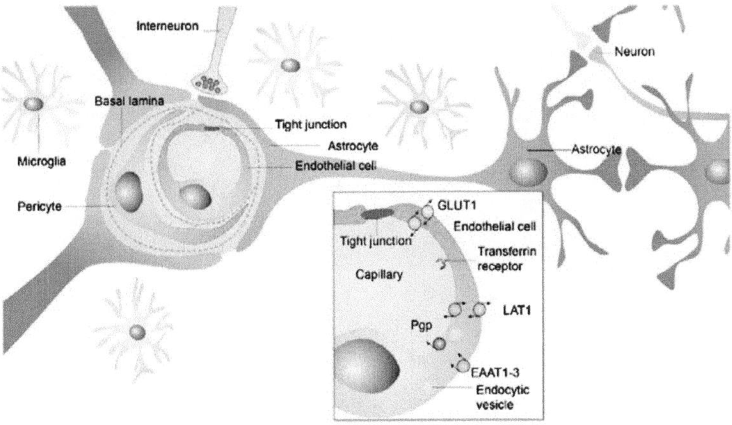


**Figure 4.1** The BBB is formed by BMVEC (see insert) that form tight junctions and express different transport systems such as Pgp, glucose transporter (GLUT1), large amino acid transporter (LAT1), excitatory amino acid transporters (EAAT1-3), transferrin receptor, and others.

the treatment of these disorders faces serious difficulty. Thus, one of the challenges of pharmaceutical research nowadays is to discover tools enabling an effective and efficacious delivery of drugs into the CNS (Fig. 4.2).

The use of nanoparticles to transport drugs across the BBB was initiated in 1990. Later, the first drug, dalargin, a hexapeptide, was transported into the brain using poly(butylcyanoacrylate) nanoparticles coated with polysorbate 80. Recently, noninvasive techniques based on colloidal carriers could represent a huge potential, since nanocarriers can protect drugs (or gene material) and deliver them across the BBB to target specific populations of brain cells.

The efficacy of the nanotechnological approach for brain targeting has been proved by several research studies. Literature contributions mainly deal with polymeric NPs, liposomes, solid lipid nanoparticles, micelles, nanogels, and dendrimers. However, if these nanocarriers are not engineered in their surface in order to take advantage of BBB transport mechanisms, they are able to target and to reach the brain to a poor extent (up to 0.1–1% of the injected dose). The ligand-based approach, one of the different

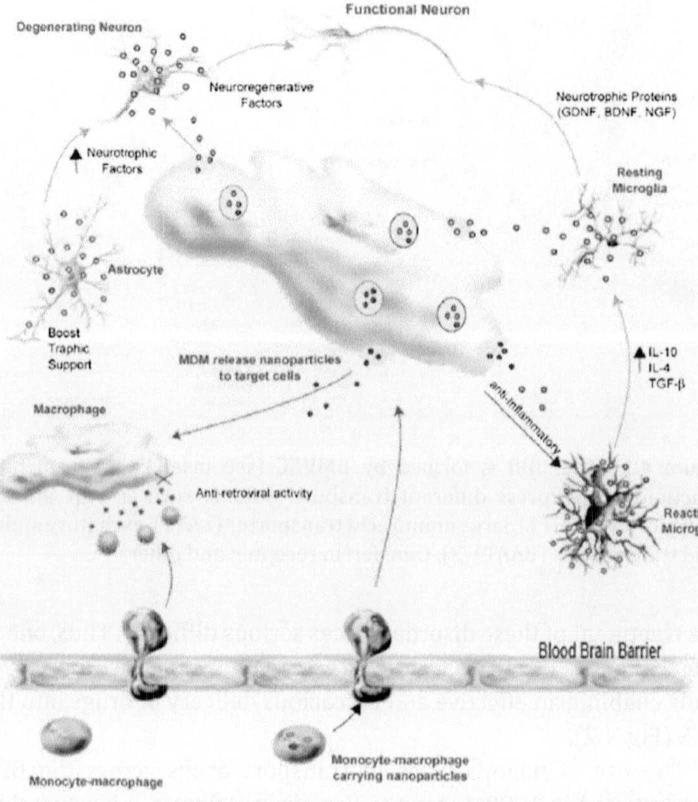


**Figure 4.2** Proposed scheme for how macrophage-based nanoparticle drug delivery could affect disease outcomes in neurodegenerative disorders. BMM would enter the brain in significant numbers carried to sites of neuroinflammation through the establishment of a chemokine gradient. Once across the BBB, macrophages would release the drug to neighboring cells, including other macrophages, microglia, astrocytes, or neurons. The nanoparticles would dissolve and release the drug that would subsequently affect neuronal viability and function, deactivation of neurotoxic inflammatory microglia, anti-retroviral responses, and astrocyte neurotrophic activities.

approaches included in NP engineering, became an interesting choice in order to achieve a more specific and selective drug delivery to the CNS, because of the possibility of promoting a direct interaction between engineered reach the brain alone, such

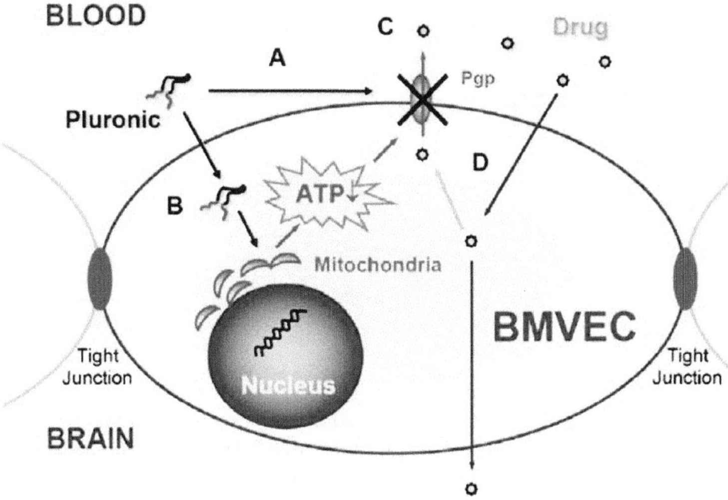


**Figure 4.3** A scheme illustrating the mechanism of Pluronic® action in BBB: (A) inhibiting PgpATPase function in cell plasma membrane; (B) inhibiting respiration in mitochondria resulting in ATP depletion. Both effects combined result in (C) inhibition of the Pgp drug efflux system and (D) transport of the drug to the brain. Reproduced with permission from *Insciences J.* 2011, 1(4), 169–193.

as rhodamine-123 and loperamide) demonstrated the ability of g7-NPs to create BBB interaction and trigger an efficacious BBB crossing, up to 10–15% of the injected dose (Fig. 4.3). In line with the overall increase in knowledge and nanotechnologies, surface engineering of nano-sized carriers now represents the cutting edge of nanomedicine, leading to the production of selectively targeted therapies based on targeted nanocarriers. In fact, achieving nanocarriers that are able to remain stable in the bloodstream, protect the drug from metabolism, and promote the long-lasting release of the drug is still a pivotal prerequisite for nanomedicine, but it is now considered as not enough. Active targeting to specific pathological cells is now the challenge for pharmaceutical nanotechnologists, who are faced with difficulties in colloidal chemistry and most of all in the characterization of the engineered nanocarriers from a technological and physiological point of view. As an example, the application of nanotechnology in brain-related

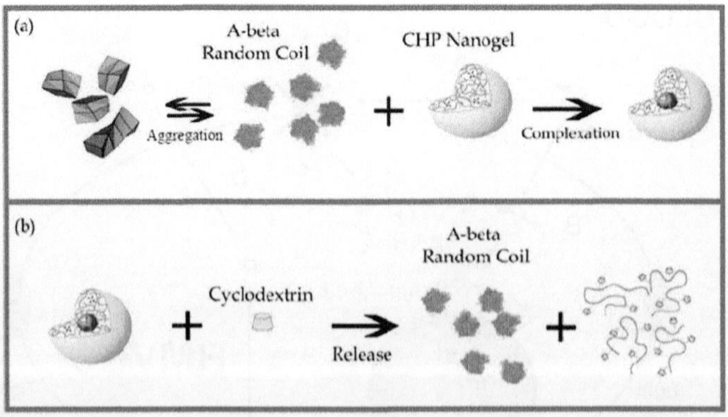


**Figure 4.4** (a) Schematic representation of the interactions between artificial nanoscale chaperon system and misfolded A$\beta$. (b) Refolded A$\beta$ monomers are released after addition of cyclodextrin.

disorders, called nanoneuromedicine, represents one of the most stimulating challenges, as well as one the most difficult, because of the presence of biological barriers (the BBB) and the great variability in BBB permeability depending on the chosen disease. Encouraging results have been obtained that demonstrate the possibility of targeting the CNS, reaching an important percentage of brain localization with respect to the injected dose. Notwithstanding these outputs, it is our opinion that in order to obtain a real update on therapy for neurological disorders based on innovative and noninvasive protocols (i.e., nanomedicine), a working group is strongly needed. The interdisciplinary competence and skills of all the experts in neurodiseases and nanotechnology (from neurobiologists to neurophysiologists, from nanotechnologists to physicians) must be shared, discussed, considered, and applied, thus opening new vistas in treatments and most of all for the correct development of the research (Fig. 4.4).

## 4.2 CNS Neuroprotective Potentials

Neurodegenerative diseases, particularly the pathogenesis of Alzheimer's disease, are caused by neurotoxicity, which mainly arises from A$\beta$ oligomers and free radicals. Protection of neurons from A$\beta$ toxicity and from oxidative stress of free radicals is possible through nanotechnology-based neuroprotective approaches, preventing amyloid oligomerization (anti-assembly strategy) and/or accumulation of A$\beta$ oligomeric species.

Fullerenes have been functionalized to serve as effective catalysts for the destruction of free radicals in injured brain tissue. Fullerene (C60) and its derivatives could be the base of neuroprotective compounds. The biological applications of fullerene, including its antioxidant and free radical scavenger potentials, are due to its kind of chemical structure that allows it to be linked (to be functionalized) to several active chemical groups in a three-dimensional orientation. The effects of carboxyfullerenes (malonic acid derivative of C60, C63[(COOH)2]3) on $A\beta42$-induced oxidative stress and neurotoxicity in cultured cortical neurons. Interestingly, the application of carboxyfullerenes blocked the $A\beta42$-induced neuronal apoptotic death. Recent findings demonstrated the anti-assembly effect of C60 hydrated fullerene (C60HyFn) on the fibrillization of $A\beta25-35$ fragment. It was demonstrated that injection of 3.6 nMol of C60HyFn to each of the brain ventricles could prevent the cognitive impairment in rats previously injected with an $A\beta25 - 35$ fragment. Fullerenes have also complete neuroprotective properties against NMDA receptor mediated neurotoxicity according to the studies of Dugan et al. NMDA receptor function is important to the neuronal mechanisms of learning and memory. Fullerenols, which are water-soluble hydroxyl-functionalized derivatives of fullerene, have shown neuroprotective properties against $A\beta42$. Presumably, the neuroprotective effect of fullerenols is due to both antioxidant reactions and inhibition of $A\beta42$-induced Ca2+ neurotoxicity. The applications of functionalized fullerene derivatives, including carboxyfullerene and hydroxyfullerene (fullerenols) and C60HyFn, are promising in the discovery of new drugs for neurodegenerative diseases; however, further research on their pharmacodynamic and pharmacokinetic properties is necessary.

Nanogels are another unique type of nanoparticle formation. These nanosized hydrogel particles are composed of a network of flexible hydrophilic cross-linked polymer strands. The hydrophic polymers can absorb large amounts of water, swelling the particles

| Nanosystem | Neuroprotective Function | Targeted AD pathology mechanism | Study Mode |
|---|---|---|---|
| Nanogels (Cholesterol bearing pullulan) | Aβ Anti- assembly (Incorporate Aβ monomers) | Oligoemrization of Aβ | In vitro (Solution and Cell Culture) |
| Fullerence ($C_{60}$)<br>Carboxyfullerence | Antioxidant<br>Aβ Anti-Assembly | Oxidative stress<br>Oligoemrization of Aβ | In vitro (cell culture) |
| C60HyFn<br>Fullerenol | Antioxidant/Maintenance of $Ca^{2+}$ homeostasis | $Ca^{++}$ influx | In vivo (Rats) |
| Dendrimers (Polyamidoamine (PAMAM)) | Aβ Anti-Assembly | Oligoemrization of Aβ<br>Aβ cell membrane toxicity | In vitro |
| Nanoceria ($CeO_2$) | Antioxidant | Oxidative Stress | In vitro |
| Gold Nanoparticles (AuNP) | Aβ Anti-Assembly | Oligoemrization of Aβ | In vitro |
| Diamondoid Derivatives (Memantime) (1-amino-3, 5-dimethyladamantane) | NMDA receptor antagonism | Glutamate excitotoxicity | In vivo (FDA approved drug) |

**Figure 4.5** Nanotechnology-suggested neuroprotective agents for the treatment of neurodegenerative diseases.

into a gel. Nano- and microgels have been found to be very useful in drug delivery and tissue regeneration because of their tissue compatibility, biodegradability, and versatility. Transport of oligonucleotides incorporated in nanogel particles across an in vitro model of the BBB was recently reported. Notably, nanogels decreased degradation of oligonucleotides during their transport in BMVEC. To further enhance delivery across the BBB, the surface of nanogels was modified by either transferrin or insulin. In vivo studies suggested that nanogels increase brain uptake of oligonucleotides while decreasing their uptake in the liver and the spleen. Overall, nanogels are promising carriers for CNS drug delivery, although they are in relatively early stages of development (Fig. 4.5).

An example for the $A\beta$ anti-assembly strategy is the design of an amphipathic nanogel that incorporates proteins and controls their folding and aggregation, similar to natural chaperons. These nanogels could incorporate $A\beta$ and inhibit the amyloidogenesis process effectively. The nanogel (hydrogel nanoparticles) was composed of cholesterol-bearing pullulan (CHP). Pullulan is a natural water-soluble polysaccharide polymer consisting of maltotriose (a trisaccharide consisting of three glucose molecules linked with 1,4 glycosidic bonds) units. Inhibiting assembly at the monomer level, this technique prevents $A\beta$ oligomerization and therefore reduces the concentration of toxic A$\beta$ oligomeric species. Recently, a significant reduction in A$\beta$42 toxicity was demonstrated in the primary cortical cell culture and microglial cell culture after using CHP nanogels.

Another potential application on neuroprotective effects has been reported for cerium oxide (CeO2) nanoparticles (nano-ceria). This is mainly due to their antioxidant properties, originating in the two oxidation–reduction (redox) states of cerium: Ce2+ and Ce4+ and the resultant oxygen vacancies. In addition to their antioxidant properties, nano-ceria protect neurons from the cytotoxic effects of A$\beta$ by modulating the intracellular signaling pathways involved in cellular death and neuroprotection.

Diamondoids are in the category of the most promising molecular building blocks in nanotechnology and, especially, nanomedicine. These particles are of macromolecular structure with globular shape and a densely packed surface. Their structure has offered them a number of biomedical potentials. Recently, a multipurpose anti-amyloid strategy was suggested for dendrimers. A$\beta$ anti-assembly strategy of dendrimers can be performed either by binding them with peptide monomers or by blocking the end of protofibrils and fibrils. Application of the modified dendrimers is a recent suggestion for this approach. Recent studies have shown that dendrimers (both conjugated and unconjugated) could shield the cell membrane from A$\beta$ membrane mediated neurotoxicity, which is due to A$\beta$ electrostatic interaction with the cell membrane. In addition, dendrimers can sequester the A$\beta$ toxic species and therefore block their pathological effects on the cell membrane. However, because of the probable toxic effect of dendrimers on cells, this method needs further investigation for in vivo application.

Further potential applications are based on diamondoid derivatives. Diamondoids and their derivatives are the basis of many varieties of antiviral and antibacterial drugs. It has been shown that a diamondoid-based drug (memantine), which is already in commercial use, slows down the progression of Alzheimer's disease. Memantine (1-amino-3, 5-dimethyladamantane), with Namenda as its commercial name, is an FDA-approved drug for the treatment of moderate to severe Alzheimer's disease. Memantine acts as a neuroprotective agent against excitotoxicity, an excessive exposure to the neurotransmitter glutamate or overstimulation of its membrane receptors, leading to neuronal injury or death. Excitotoxic neuronal cell death is mediated in part by overactivation of N-methyl-d-aspartate (NMDA)-type glutamate receptors. Nevertheless, NMDA receptor activity is also essential for normal neuronal function. This means that potential neuroprotective agents that block virtually all NMDA receptor activity will very likely have unacceptable clinical side effects. Memantine preferentially blocks excessive NMDA receptor activity without disrupting normal activity. Although memantine is already approved by FDA for the treatment of Alzheimer's disease, studies are under way for other diamondoid derivatives which could have stronger neuroprotective and, possibly, regenerative capability, as well as for their application for the treatment of diseases related to glutamatergic dysfunction.

## 4.3 Nanocarriers and CNS-Targeted Drug Delivery

Targeted drug delivery with implementation of nanomedicine is having a significant impact on the diagnosis and treatment of neurodegenerative diseases. The use of biocompatible nanoparticles to facilitate therapeutic agents to traverse the BBB has been extensively researched in the past decade. Nanoengineered encapsulation has been shown to be a promising therapeutic strategy for CNS regeneration.

- **Nanoencapsulation drug delivery**

  Targeted and time release of drugs can be processed as drug conjugation with antibodies and other macromolcules, microencapsulation, and nanoparticles. The biodegradable polymeric nanoparticles are offering an alternative for the transport of a wide range of drugs in a way that can change the delivery process from free-flowing circulation to targeted release in a chosen controlled environment. These nanocarriers are being formulated with various physicochemical properties and can be made with safe materials, including synthetic biodegradable polymers, lipids, and polysaccharides. The nanoparticles can

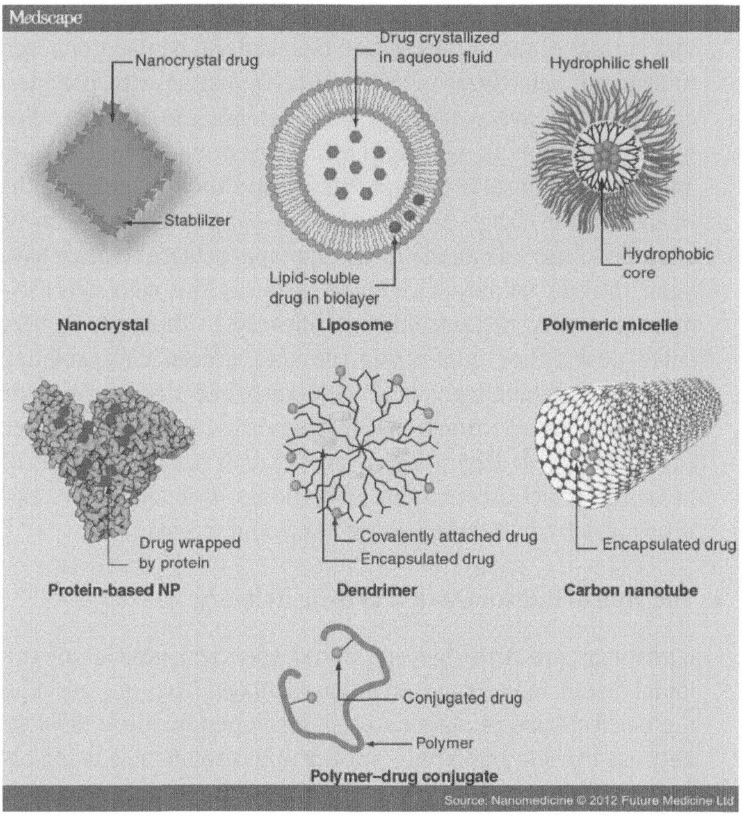


**Figure 4.6** Examples of nanoparticles and nanoencapsulation types (Orive et al., *Nat. Rev. Neurosci.* 10, 682, 2009. Reproduced with permission from Nanoencapsulation Methods.

also be targeted to certain cell types by adding a molecular recognition function to the particle which binds to or enters the targeted cells (Fig. 4.6). Nanosized particles can deliver drugs in novel ways. While conjugation with the nanoparticle carrier material offers many delivery possibilities, an alternative is to enclose the drug inside a protective shell, giving a more complete separation between the delivery vehicle and the therapeutic agent. With nanoencapsulation formulations, release of the drug can take place gradually through diffusion, dissolution, or biodegradation, or an engineered nanocapsule can be used to deliver the drug to a selected environment. The surface of the encapsulation material can be functionalized to attach it selectively to targeted cells, just as with polymer-conjugated delivery systems. Drug release can be controlled by pH, or by functionalizing the surfaces of nanoparticles with antibodies to localize targeted tissue and then stimulating the release of the drugs. Even the body's own blood cells can be adapted to carry a nanomedicine: nanoparticulate steroids have been introduced into red blood cells; as the cells die their natural deaths, the steroids are released in the body in very small doses, thus minimizing the side effects. Encapsulation strategies include polymers with absorbed drugs, dendritic molecules, or coordination compounds with drugs bounded covalently, or weakly attached, artificial, or natural micelles or liposome vesicles containing nano-doses of insoluble or toxic drugs which can be selectively released on targets.

- **The role of liposomes in CNS drug delivery**

Liposomes are artificially prepared spherical vesicles of colloidal dimensions composed of a lipid bilayer. They are, perhaps, the earliest type of nanomaterial developed for drug delivery. Because of their amphiphilic nature and resemblance to biological membrane, they contain an inner and outer hydrophobic core for entrapping and delivering the hydrophilic drugs. The physicochemical properties of liposomes enhance their specificity, and they show excellent penetration and diffusion properties. Overall, they are nontoxic, being biocompatible and biodegradable. Liposomes are tailored with several polymers to reduce recognition by the reticuloendothelial system, and thereby to prolong circulation and retention time. Several varieties of liposomes used to transport drugs over the BBB include small unilamellar vesicles, multilamellar vesicles, polyethylene glycol (PEG)-coated liposomes, PEGylated ligand/antibody-bearing immunoliposomes, and stimuli-sensitive liposomes. The coating of liposomes with hydrophilic polymers such as PEG, poly(alkylcyanoacrylates), poloxamines, poloxamers, and polysaccharides have been proposed as an interesting alternative that can reduce opsonization and prolong circulation time, reduce drug side effects, and thus enhance targeted brain delivery. The circulation half-life of PEGylated liposomes is around 50 hours in humans. It has been shown that PEGylated liposomes can accumulate more rapidly in the brain when the BBB is compromised. Artificial liposomes are another example of encapsulated drugs, coated with a biodegradable polymer to which antibodies can be attached. The antibodies are recognized by the brain capillary receptors, which mediate their passage through the BBB. Once inside the central nervous system, the liposomes release their contents.

There have been intensive research studies on evaluating liposomes for CNS drug delivery. In a recent study, the researchers exploited the BBB transit of phagocytic immune cells by loading them with tailored liposomes containing serotonin, a neurotransmitter in the central and peripheral nervous system. These liposomes were in the range of 100–250 nm and are unusually not hydrophilic, do not have a neutral membrane, and are not of ultra size. This results in the efficient uptake by phagocytic cells (monocytes and neutrophils) and increased circulation period, and apart from undergoing rapid clearance in the liver and the spleen, these phagocytic cells will transport the drug across the BBB, with the drug then being released from the cells in the brain. Intravenous administration of these negatively charged serotonin liposomes exhibited two times higher uptake than free serotonin, which otherwise does not transit the BBB. PEGylated immunoliposomes, containing genetically engineered monoclonal antibodies directed to insulin or transferring receptors, have been successfully used as carriers for gene replacement therapy in the Parkinson model. Recent findings reported potential applications of transferrin-conjugated liposomes in targeting post-ischemic brain endothelium. The expression of this transferrin receptor, which is necessary to deliver iron across the BBB, is expected to be increased in certain pathologies, for instance after a stroke. One of the challenges in using liposomes for drug delivery is their lack of stability. Polymer-caged liposomes are one of the recent methods used for stabilizing liposomes within a polymer which can fall apart and trigger drug release when taken into cells.

Similar to liposomes, polymersomes have been actively investigated for therapeutic targeting and delivery, as they can be used to encapsulate and deliver drugs, proteins, and genetic material, in addition to being a potential tool for cell tracking.

- **Applications based on polymeric micelles**

Polymeric micelles have been well suited for drug delivery purposes with their inherent structures and modifiable properties (association, morphology, size, and stability) that make them encapsulate considerable amounts of water-insoluble drugs and prevent premature drug release and degradation. These micelles are usually formed in solutions of amphiphilic block copolymers with sizes varying from ca. 10 to 100 nm. They have a core–shell structure (e.g., poly(caprolactone), poly(D,L-lactide), poly(propylene glycol) (PPG), and shell blocks (PEG)). The most widely studied block copolymer classes are poly(propylene oxide), poly(L-amino acid)s, and poly(ester)s. These three classes of block copolymers are under current research in which formulation techniques have been applied to some of the most challenging molecules in the pharmaceutical industry. These three copolymer classes have shown the ability to attenuate toxicities. Their nanoscopic structure masks the delivered drug from interactions with untargeted cells and serum proteins, and hence protects encapsulated substances from degradation and metabolism. Several clinical trials are under way to evaluate polymeric micelles for enhancing anticancer drug delivery and improving the therapeutic efficacy of active pharmaceutical ingredients.

Recently, micelles of Pluronic block copolymers (PEG-b-PPG-b-PEG) have been used as carriers for CNS drug delivery. Drugs can be incorporated in micelle carriers by covalent or ionic bonding to the micelle-forming materials. In the central nervous system, these micelles were conjugated with either polyclonal antibodies against brain 2-glycoprotein or insulin as targeting moieties. Both antibody- and insulin-vectorized micelles were shown to deliver a drug or a fluorescent probe to the brain in vivo. Recent studies have shown a considerable increase in neuroleptic activity of a drug (haloperidol) solubilized in the targeted micelles compared to a free drug.

Polymer micelles have demonstrated some success, especially with incorporating block copolymers, to help evade elimination by the immune system.

- **The role of nanocarriers in CNS-targeted drug therapy**

Acetylcholine nanocarrier: Acetylcholine is an organic molecule that acts as a neurotransmitter. It has functions both in the peripheral nervous system (PNS) and in the central nervous system (CNS) and is the only neuromodulator used in the motor division of the somatic nervous system. Its receptors have very high binding constants. In the peripheral nervous system, acetylcholine activates muscles and is a major neurotransmitter in the autonomic nervous system. In the central nervous system, acetylcholine and the associated neurons form a neurotransmitter system, the cholinergic system, which tends to cause inhibitory actions. Recent studies on acetylcholine nanocarrier in Alzheimer's disease were demonstrated in the delivery of acetylcholine to lysosomes in the brain of AD mice mode through low doses of single-wall carbon nanotubes (SWCNs).

Chelator nanocarriers: Recently chelator nanoparticle systems have shown to be a potential therapeutic approach to prevent and treat neurodegenerative diseases. It has been shown that the use of nanoparticles for target transport of chelators could provide more effective and safer therapeutics. Some studies have shown that nanoparticles have the potential to transfer chelators in and out brain, thus effectively preventing metal-associated oxidative damage. This novel approach of chelation will provide not only a useful means of treating neurodegerative diseases, but also insights into the pathophysiological mechanisms of the disease. It may also show utility in all iron-mediated neurodegenerative diseases such as Friedreich's ataxia, Parkinson's disease, and Hallervorden-Spatz syndrome.

Recent studies on Alzheimer's disease (AD) have shown that metal chelation strategy may substantially decrease both the extracellular oxidative stress and A$\beta$ aggregation, and therefore slow down the progression of the disease.

One of the efficient chelator nanoparticle systems (CNPS) can be produced with the conjugation of desferrioxamine (DFO), an FDA-approved iron chelator, with nanoparticles. The formation can be formed through an amido bond between a primary amino group in the chelator and a carboxyl group on the nanoparticle surface. The advantages of using a nanoparticle system for drug delivery are evident in the feasibility of carrying iron chelators across the BBB. For iron chelation to be effective, the chelators must be capable of leaving the brain with the corresponding complexed metal ions. It has been shown that the iron chelating CNPS was able to traverse the BBB in the reverse direction by preferential adsorption of Apo A-I and, thereby, removal through the LDL transport system. There is an obvious reduction in the inherent toxicity of the chelators after conjugation with nanoparticles. Recent studies on iron chelator have demonstrated some therapeutic benefits for patients with Alzheimer's disease. Recently, chelation DFO has reportedly been found to significantly slow the progression of the disease in one clinical trial. Its therapy promotes iron excretion and has led to great improvements in the quality and duration of the life of patients who suffer from $\beta$ thalassemia and other refractory anemias. However, DFO is poorly absorbed by the gastrointestinal tract and rapidly degrades after administration. Therefore, it requires long subcutaneous administration to be given parenterally, as a continuous subcutaneous infusion or as a continuous intravenous infusion, to yield significant iron excretion. Moreover, some studies show that DFO does not easily penetrate the BBB. However, it has been shown that some penetration may occur because of a compromised BBB via lesion sites.

There are three advantages to this approach. First, the chelators need not be lipophilic to cross the BBB. Second, the lipophilic character of the chelator no longer contributes to potential toxicity. And third, hydrophilic hexadentate iron chelators with large molecular weights may be used, as previously demonstrated with nanoparticle technology. Moreover, it was suggested that the inherent toxicity of the chelators is obviously decreased after conjugation with nanoparticles.

The carboxyl-functionalized polystyrene nanoparticle is another synthesized nanoparticle chelator conjugate (Nano-N2PY) which may reduce the toxicity of the chelation strategy by decreasing the lipophilicity of the chelators. The conjugate is also capable of transporting metal chelators across the BBB, without disrupting the metal binding feature of the chelator.

Another FDA-approved metal chelator examined for Wilson's disease is d-penicillamine. This copper chelator is capable of disolubilizing A$\beta$42.

The nanoparticles used in CNPS formation contained 1,2-dioleoyl-snglycero-3-phosphoethanolamine-N-[4-(p-maleimidophenyl)- butyramide] (MPB-PE) and pyridyldithiopropionyl phosphoethanolamine (PDP-PE).

The study demonstrated that the copper-chelating CNPS was able to traverse the BBB in spite of its highly hydrophilic properties, and no changes were evident in the BBB permeability integrity.

Curcuminoid nanocarriers: It has been discovered that curcuminoid, a therapeutic agent which is the active ingredient of the yellow spice turmeric, is an effective treatment for Alzheimer's disease. It has been demonstrated that this agent acts as an antioxidant, anti-inammatory, and antiamyloid assembly. For the transport of this unstable therapeutic agent through the BBB, poly n-butylcyanoacrylate (PnBCA) nanocapsules coated with apolipoprotein E3 (APoE-3) have been used for the crossover.

Antioxidant agent nanocarriers: Nanopaticles based on solid lipids have developed as modern nanofabricated extensions of early lipid emulsion drug formulations. Much improvement in the drug delivery of antioxidant agents has been made by using nanocarriers based on solid lipid nanoparticles (SLNs). Three types of SLNs have been developed for drug delivery and therapy: solid lipid nanoparticles, nanostructured lipid carriers, and lipid drug conjugates. These nanodrugs have been formulated with the aim of overcoming some of the difficulties of liposomes. The advantages of using these nanocarriers are evident in the feasibility of carrying ferulic acid (FA) [3-(4-hydroxy- 3-methoxyphenyl)-2-propenoic acid], which is a highly antioxidant phenolic compound, thus improving drug stability within fluids and making intracellular targeting feasible. FA may cause increased cell viability in exposing neuroblastoma cells to A42 oligomers, because it highly affects the normalized mitochondrial membrane potential, ROS production, and cytochrom C release. Using nanocarriers overcomes some of the difficulties of liposomes.

- **The role of gene nanocarrier therapy**

Gene therapy for nerve regeneration has been a promising strategy for many years. Accompanying the genetic material with a carrier may protect it from biological obstacles, like cell membrane charge and enzymatic degradation. Viral vectors have been employed so far in most of the gene therapy studies for neurodegenerative diseases. However, because of the size limitation of genetic inserts through viral vectors and possible associated health risks, the use of nanoparticles as nonviral gene carriers has become the focus of attention in recent studies. Using such alternative nonviral vectors has the advantage of minimizing the enzymatic degradation of genetic materials. Recent findings on polymeric, ceramic, and amino-terminated, organically modified silica (ORMOSIL) nanoparticles demonstrated the potential of ORMOSIL nanoparticles for bioconjugation and in vivo gene transfection. The surface modification of ORMOSIL with various functional groups plays a critical role providing novel properties and functionalities for these nontoxic nanoparticles. The surface properties of silica particles play a significant role in the interaction of the particles with bioenvironments and determine the cellular uptake and cytotoxicity of the resulting particles. The colloidal stability of the particles can be increased in such resultant functional groups. They can also be utilized for conjugation to different biomoieties for targeting specific gene/drug delivery to various cancerous cells. Moreover, being functionalized with amino groups for DNA binding, the ORMOSIL nanoparticles are found to be appropriate gene vectors in in vivo brain therapy and for therapeutic regulation of neural stem cells. On the leading edge of research, nanomaterials can provide active signaling cues for guided axon growth in brain regeneration therapies.

Recently encapsulated delivery of cells genetically engineered to produce ciliary neurotrophic factor (CNTF) has been evaluated for the treatment of ALS in phase I and II trials on 12 patients. CNTF was delivered in the cerebrospinal fluid of nine patients and persisted for up to 20 weeks in two patients. No adverse side effects were reported in the patients.

Nanoengineered biomaterials and structures for protection and regeneration of injuries in the CNS are being investigated for potential clinical applications. In the meantime, research on nanoengineered scaffolds for brain regeneration is producing promising results.

## 4.4 Applications Based on Cell-Mediated Drug Delivery

An alternative approach to CNS antiretroviral drug delivery is to administer a drug systemically in conjunction with transient disruption of the BBB as molecules could be allowed passage where otherwise they would not. However, BBB disruption may lead to serious complications because of possible access of unwanted blood components to the CNS. A number of nanotechnology-based explorative strategies for crossing the BBB have been recently developed for getting antiretroviral drugs into the brain on the basis of BBB disruption, development of NPs with increased BBB permeability, and uptake by brain microvessel endothelial cells (BMVECs) via adsorptive-mediated transcytosis and cell-mediated delivery. Another novel approach is based on the disruption of the BBB with electromagnetic interference (EMI) in the form of amplitude-modulated (AM)/frequency-modulated (FM) waves that leads to altering the permeability of BMVECs. Recent findings have shown that implementing EMI in the disruption of human BMVECs increases permeability to antiretroviral-containing NPs across the cell monolayer. It was also demonstrated that square AM waves had the strongest effect by increasing permeability to NPs (polymeric NPs and solid lipid NPs)) by more than 14-fold, while having almost no effect on the permeability of the free drug.

Not only dead bacteria but also live cells can be used to deliver drugs. Tumor cells create inflammation signals which attract white blood cells. Researchers use a clever strategy to recruit monocytes into tumor tissue as Trojan horses. First, the monocytes are induced to engulf specially coated gold nanoshells. These white cells are released to invade the tumor, and then the phagocytized gold nanodots are heated by photoinduction. The monocytes become kamikaze cells, destroying the surrounding tumor cells.

The role of cell-mediated drug delivery has shown promising results in the treatment of neuroinfalammatory diseases. On the basis of clear connections existing between inflammation and neurodegeneration, it has been shown that biological processes causing inflammatory responses are common links to many other neurodegenerative diseases. Recent findings reported highly divergent diseases, such as stroke, ALS, PD, AD, PD, HAD, and spongiform encephalopathies or prion-mediated neurodegeneration, which have in common an inflammatory component as their inflammation processes are characterized by extensive recruitment of leukocytes (neutrophils and monocytes) engaged in attempts to eliminate the invader along with clearance of damaged tissue.

The ability of nanoparticles to affect penetration of the BBB is an important aspect of their effectiveness for neurodegenerative disorders. Great progress has been made on comprehending the role of mononuclear phagocytes (MPs) in immunity and most notably in the cell-mediated CNS drug delivery in neurodegenerative diseases. MPs as monocytes and macrophages can be used to uptake, transport, and deliver NPs containing antiretroviral drugs to the brain. As CNS inflammatory infiltrates are complex and multifaceted, the MP and T cell elements of innate immunity set up a cascade, migrating toward the site of inflammation through the diapedesis and chemataxis processes. The cascade may further affect the activation and recruitment of the adaptive immune system and ultimately tissue destruction.

The uptake of nanoparticles by MPs is affected by size, shape, charge, and surface modification. As such, the NPs are tracked to secondary lysosomes within the cells. Inside a secondary lysosome, the NPs will release the encapsulated drug once they encounter a low pH environment. NPs such as dendrimers, gelatin NPs, polymer blend NPs, lipid-drug liposomes, and nanocrystals are ideally suited for cell-mediated drug delivery.

The role of metal NPs (such as gold and silver) in immunity and most notably in the CNS has been extensively researched. Also, their interaction with proteins such as amyloid in Alzheimer's disease and synuclein in Parkinson's disease has been investigated. In the past century, a great deal of their use has been realized in imaging, and bioassays are now being implemented for possible use in neurodegenerative and antiretroviral HIV therapies.

Functionalized gold nanoparticles (AuNPs), which possess special optical properties and the potential to be used as an ideal colorimetric sensor, can be used as the basis for drug carriers and DNA/gene delivery, which shows promising results in the treatment of neurodegerative diseases. Gold NPs are proven to convert inactive drugs into potent viral inhibitors, as these NPs can easily be conjugated to SDC-1721, a fragment of the potent HIV inhibitor TAK-779. This provides conjugated SDC-1721 with inhibitory effect on HIV infection. Another interesting drug-free method of viral inhibition is the interaction of silver NPs with HIV in a size-dependent manner that inhibits infection in vitro. Such interaction may occur through preferential binding to HIV-1 gp120 glycoprotein knobs. However, the interaction of metal NPs with viruses has not been yet largely explored, and yet more work needs to be done on this investigation.

As the aggregated structure of SOD1 in motor neurons is a key feature of the pathology of ALS, a simple and sensitive colorimetric assay employing the SOD1 protein conjugated on the surface of gold nanoparticles was effectively used as a sensor for the detection of structural evolution of SOD1 aggregates. This proposed sensor system is based on highly sensitive changes in the local dielectric environment of SOD1-AuNPs that alters the surface plasmon resonance spectra, correlated with even small amount of SOD1 aggregation, which can give quantitative information in tracking the structural evolution of SOD1 aggregates and provides the prospective potential for definitive diagnosis of ALS. On the other hand, utilization of nano-flow liquid chromatography coupled with several advanced imaging techniques was also shown to enable the discovery of biomarkers in ALS patients.

In line with NPs, another promising approach to CNS delivery is protein conjugation with Pluronic block copolymers. It has been shown that HRP modified with Pluronic P85 and L121 displayed increased BBB permeability compared to native HRP. In vivo studies demonstrated a fourfold increase in the rates of modified HRP entry into the brain compared with unmodified protein, which resulted in almost a twofold increase in its brain accumulation. This technology has shown to be promising for improving the delivery of protein-based diagnostic and therapeutic agents to the brain. Another application of NP delivery is siRNA, which recently attracted some attention and holds high potential as a novel class of therapeutics. However, its low stability and need for intracellular delivery prevented its clinical translation.

In the last decade, research in nanomedicine has strongly focused on the use of specific ligands (e.g., antibodies, peptides, substrates of receptors) to be conjugated onto the surface of NPs and liposomes, thus enabling nanocarriers to specifically target cell populations or to cross virtually impermeable barriers, such as the BBB. Nanomedicine has transformed modern-day therapeutics through its novel opportunities in biosensing, imaging, diagnosis, and therapy including antiretroviral treatment and so on. Some important factors should be considered when approaching nanomedicine, such as its development in comparison with other innovative approaches and its application to the most difficult-to-treat diseases and neurological disorders.

The rapid progress in nanomedicine has opened new opportunities for the development of more effective therapies which are beginning to produce results in the form of clinical trials and emergence of new approved therapies in healthcare practice.

## 4.5 CNS Nano-Based Diagnostic Approaches

One of the most straightforward applications of nanoparticles is enhancing medical images. Nanoparticles have been used to capture and enhance images since the development of silver halide photography, but the new nanoscience has developed much more powerful and selective particles, which exploit the unique optical features found at the nanoscale. Nanoparticles are being used to enhance medical imaging for diagnosis with many modalities, including X-ray, computed tomography (CT), magnetic resonance (MRI), optical coherence tomography (OCT), wide-field optical and photoacoustic fluorescent microscopy, and infrared (IR) and ultrasound imaging.

Contrast enhancement of images is important in the diagnosis of soft tissue disorders and diseases, and particularly useful in the diagnosis of cancer and neurological diseases. In addition to contrast enhancement, nanoparticles can be functionalized to target specific cells, thus highlighting tumors, inflammation, endocrine disorders, and other type of diseases. In this respect, nanoparticles can be used in a manner similar to nuclear medicine's pharmaceutical agents, but without the disadvantages of radioactivity. It has been shown that multiple properties may be easily combined within one nanoparticle for detection with several imaging techniques or for delivery of drugs or therapeutic actions. Integrating different imaging enhancement capabilities in nanoparticles enhances the use of imaging modalities that are complementary to each other, such as MRI and optical imaging.

Conjugation compounds containing gadolinium (Gd) and radioisotopes in a dendritic molecular structure have been developed for CT imaging. However, in such systems, only a relatively small number of heavy atoms may be delivered to the vicinity of the target tissues. Nanoparticle contrast agents offer an alternative to the drawbacks of chemical agents, even those encapsulated in liposomes or polymers. In order to enhance an X-ray image, an agent must deliver a detectable number of heavy atoms into the imaged tissues without toxic effects. This issue can be overcome by using nanoparticles made of heavy metal compounds encapsulated in gold shells, or even using hollow gold nanoparticles. By functionalizing proteins with the thiol group, gold particles can be coated with selectively binding antigens, antibodies, or target compounds for receptors on the surfaces of cells. By targeting receptors, gold nanoparticles can be made to enhance the X-ray image to enable it to be detected by many orders of magnitude.

There have been a wide range of neuroimaging molecular imaging methods that have shown potential contribution in the diagnosis of neurological complications associated with neurodegenerative disorders such as positron emission tomography (PET), single-photon emission computed tomography (SPECT), magnetic resonance imaging (MRI), and computed tomography (CT). These methods have the potential to identify underlying neurological processes involved in disease progression. These conventional modalities are often used to supplement clinical and neurological examinations for the diagnosis of a variety of degenerative disorders of the CNS including HIV-1-associated cognitive impairments. In particular, MRI, diffusion tensor imaging (DTI), and CT can delineate the structural and metabolic effects of diseases and can easily depict brain atrophy. The role of functional imaging has shown greater value compared with the other methods as it is a more sensitive indicator of neurological disease, and can reveal abnormalities before structural atrophy or focal CNS lesions are visible when subtle clinical abnormalities are seen on examination. For early detection of brain dysfunction, magnetic resonance spectroscopic imaging has emerged as an effective approach based on quantitating neuronal loss performed with conventional resonance imagers.

On the other hand, clinical and laboratory examination cannot be used independently as a measure of disease diagnosis or staging. This all points to the need for developing advanced diagnostic approaches for detecting early functional abnormalities before morphological changes occur.

The development of nano-based contrast agents has attracted a phenomenal amount of research, particularly for applications in molecular imaging. Nano-based contrast agents such as fluorescent dye-doped silica nanoparticles, quantum dots, gold nanoparticles, and iron oxide nanoparticles have overcome many of the limitations of conventional contrast agents (organic dyes) such as poor photostability, low quantum yields, and low in vitro and in vivo stability. The role of nano-based contrast agents in MRI played an important role in the diagnosis of neurodegenerative diseases. MRI imaging can be intensified by solutions or dispersions of dendritic macromolecules designed for biocompatibility, or by chelating paramagnetic (gadolinium) or supermagnetic (iron or manganese) ions. The exploitation of quantum resonance effects on the nanoscale is a logical extension of the use of contrast agents for signal intensification agents for MRI imaging. It has been shown that quantum nanodots are powerful and versatile in a wide range of modalities from X-ray to ultraviolet fluorescence and visible and infrared imaging. Nanoparticles that have strong optical sensitivity in the near-infrared (NIR) and visible regions (500–800 nm) can be used for contrast enhancement for many optical biomedical imaging techniques important in cellular imaging and diagnosis, including photoacoustic imaging, optoacoustic tomography, laser optoacoustic imaging system, optical coherence tomography, and confocal and fluorescence microscopy. In addition to diagnostic tool and innovative therapies, nanoparticle imaging agents are being used as probes to understand biological processes at the molecular level. Nanoparticles with UV and visible resonance have been synthesized for use as imaging agents to study cell signaling pathways by biofunctionalization of metal, semiconductor, ceramic, and dye-doped silica nanoparticles. These particles can be applied as imaging probes to detect signaling pathway components and cellular response to signals in inflammatory cells. The application of magnetic nanoparticles for MRI enhancement can selectively target and highlight aspects of cellular metabolism. Recent studies reported potential contribution of superparamagnetic iron oxide (SPIO) and ultrasmall superparamagnetic iron oxide (USPIO) nanoparticles as MR contrast agents for monitoring the tracking of particles and cells and characterizing particle delivery in the central nervous system.

### 4.5.1 *Proposed in vitro Nanodiagnostic Approaches*

One of the potential in vitro nano-based approaches for the detection of molecular biomarkers in the CNS is the localized surface plasmon resonance (LSPR) nanosensor, which is based on the singular optical properties of triangular silver nanoparticles (AgNPs). In this method, surface resonance is used in quantum dot nanoparticles to enhance medical imaging and diagnosis. The technique is based on detecting the changes in the nanoparticles' external nanoenvironment which leads to a change in the refractive index of the surrounding magnetic field and subsequently changes the AgNPs' $\lambda_{max}$ that could be detectable via spectroscopy.

It has been shown that optical measurements at the nanoscale can utilize SPR effects, which are extremely sensitive to the absorbed layers of molecules, and can even detect single molecules if the quantum resonance well is suitably designed. SPR is recently being used in a number of in vitro and in vivo biosensing applications for clinical and pathological diagnostics. Advanced studies have shown that magnetic nanoparticles can be combined with SPR to create multifunctional diagnostic sensors that combine magnetic separation and concentration with optical reporting. One of the recent applications of the SPR nanosensor has been reported in studying the drug interactions with the target molecules in Alzheimer's disease.

DNA–nanoparticle conjugates, known as the bio-barcode assays, are another potential nano-based approach which aims to detect the concentrations of protein biomarkers. This method is based on conjugating AuNPs that match the specific antibody of the target biomarker with hundreds of DNA barcodes. The detected signal could be additionally amplified by the polymerase chain reaction (PCR) technique. Recent investigations have shown another application based on the detection of the transformed signal by two-photon Rayleigh scattering. In this technique, AuNP conjugates with anti-tau antibody to detect tau proteins at 1 pg/ml level in 35 minutes, which makes it a fast, specific, and ultrasensitive nanosensor for detecting tau protein.

### 4.5.2 *Proposed in vivo Nanodiagnostic Approaches*

Magnetic nanoparticle probes are becoming an emerging class of novel contrast and tracking agents for medical imaging. With variations in the size, coating thickness, surface chemistry, and targeting ligands, these nanoparticle probes can be tailored to target specific organs, cells, or even molecular markers of various diseases. The use of iron oxide nanoparticles as MRI contrast agents has been widely researched in the recent decades. There have been several studies that employed magnetic nanoparticles because of their specific molecular, biological, and some multifunctional features to characterize the inflammatory process in neurodegenerative disorders and atherosclerosis. Recent applications have shown that the combination of MRI and contrast agents can greatly enhance the possibility of depicting the vascular system, inflamed tissue as in arthritis, tumor angiogenesis, atherosclerotic plaques, and the breakdown of the BBB related to pathologies in neurodegenerative diseases. In neurodegenerative disorders, recent studies have shown inflammatory markers in affected neural tissues of ALS patients. Several USPIO-based contrast agents have been investigated in order to characterize acute and chronic diseases with the ongoing process of inflammation.

Our recent studies on the ALS rat model using MRI revealed T2-weighted hyperintensities in the brainstem, rubrospinal tract, and vagus motor nuclei with prominent lateral ventricle and cerebral aqueduct enlargements. Notably, with CLUSPIO antibodies against CD4, MRI revealed infiltrations of helper T cells in the interbrain regions that were shown to be correlated with the foci of neurodegeneration in these areas, not observed in the WT animals (Fig. 4.7).

Recent investigations have reported the application of USPIO nanoparticles as MRI contrast agents for in vivo detection of amyloid plaques in the brain of the transgenic mouse model. In both these studies, $A\beta$ peptide was conjugated to the nanoparticle in order to detect amyloid plaques. This technique is claimed to be minimally invasive especially if the MRI enhancement agent (nanoparticles) is injected intravenously rather than intra-arterially. However, since the $A\beta$ plaques are targeted in the above-mentioned techniques, the technique could not be useful for very early diagnosis of AD. This is because the $A\beta$ plaque formation is observed in later, more advanced stages of the disease. Therefore, the application of this technique in the detection of AD may be limited to the confirmation of established AD pathology in dementia patients, and monitoring therapeutic efficacy for those drugs that are aimed to reduce $A\beta$ plaques.

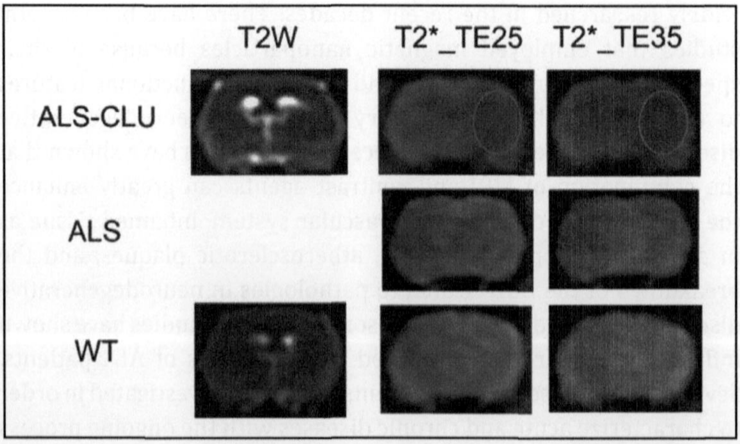


**Figure 4.7** MRI of the brain of the ALS rat treated with CLUSPIO (ALS-CLU) as compared to the MRI of the ALS rat without CLUSPIO injection (ALS) and of the wild-type rat (WT). T2W protocol reveals the dilated ventricles in the ALS model (images in the left column). T2* protocol reveals the hypointensities (note regions delimited by ellipsoids) 12 allegedly caused by CLUSPIO seen with time to echo (TE) 25 ms (middle column) and further augmented with TE 35 ms (right column).

#### 4.5.2.1 Nano-based optical imaging

Intensive efforts have been going on for the development of a class of multimodal contrast agents which can combine magnetic resonance imaging (MRI) and optical imaging. One of the recently developed optical imaging techniques is surface-enhanced coherent anti-Stokes Raman scattering (SECARS) microscopy. The potential of this imaging modality is highlighted by the drastic signal enhanced in the vicinity of nanoparticles, as molecules trapped in nanoparticle junctions, that can increase the detection sensitivity reaching the single-molecule level, which makes it a promising high-resolution imaging technique.

Another recently growing approach for in vivo detection of molecular biomarkers is optical imaging through special near-infrared NIR fluorescent contrast agents. Because of the long wavelength, the scattered light from these contrast agents can penetrate through biological tissues. Promising applications based on these methods have been introduced.

#### 4.5.2.2 SECARS microscopy

SECARS microscopy is a newly developed innovative imaging technique based on the combination of a third-order nonlinear Raman optical effect with surface enhancement Raman scattering (SERS). Earlier published demonstrations of SECARS microscopy showed the feasibility of this method for enhanced detection sensitivity in biological systems.

The method involves the input of two fields of frequencies, $\omega P$ and $\omega S(\omega P > \omega S)$. Two photons of the pump field at frequency $\omega P$ interact with a single photon of the Stokes field at frequency $\omega S$ to create an output field with a frequency of $\omega AS = 2\omega P - \omega S$. In this process, the two input frequencies are set so that $\omega P - \omega S$ is near a Raman transition. Consequently, a large signal is produced at the anti-Stokes frequency with the same average excitation power compared with spontaneous Raman signal. The signal is further improved by aggregation of the nanoparticles in the presence of biological molecules, as molecules trapped in nanoparticle junctions. The main strength of this technique lies in the fact that it can image the native and unaltered state of the samples or the nanoparticles without the additional labeling or fluorescent marker. This is important since the marker may change the behavior of the, e.g., metallic/organic state of the nanoparticles in the cells.

In recent studies, SECARS microscopy has been exploited in nanodiagnostic applications on monitoring USPIO uptakes in neurodegenerative disorder systems (ALS). In line with the MRI findings, ex vivo SECARS experiments performed on CLUSPIO i.v. injected brain sections taken from ALS transgenic rat model showed marked signal enhancement in specific pathological regions, particularly in the midbrain and the brainstem known to be infiltrated by helper T cells. The prominent bands that showed significant enhancement observed in the high-frequency region were around 2845 and 2875 $cm^{-1}$, which are typical bands for fatty acids dominated by valence vibrations of C-H2 groups (Fig. 4.8). The bands from 2700 to 3500 $cm^{-1}$ are correlated to cholesterol ester (cholesteryl palmitate), triacylglyceride (glyceryl palmitate), phosphatidic acid, and sphingomyelin. Significant enhancements were also observed in

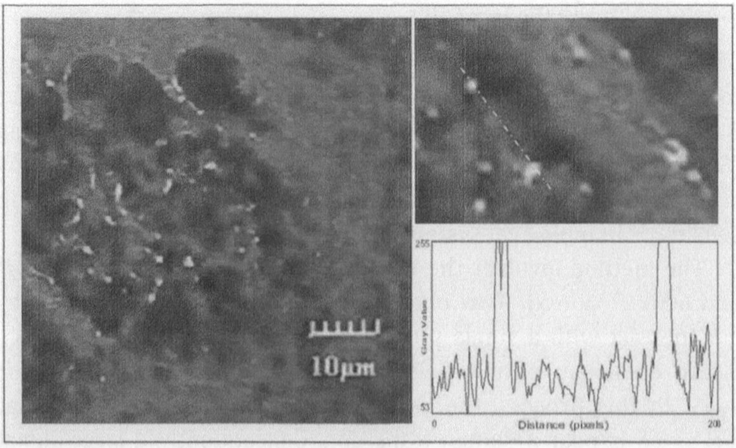


**Figure 4.8** SECARS image of brain tissue from CLUSPIO-treated ALS rats, taken at 2850 cm$^{-1}$. The corresponding cross-section profile shows the intensity enhancement along the indicated line.

the fingerprint region around 1660–1675 cm$^{-1}$, which is correlated to unsaturated fatty acids and to the steroid ring of cholesterol (Fig. 4.9). In this study, the SECARS enhancement was correlated to the lipid iron accumulation in the inflammatory cells or from regions with perturbed sphingolipid metabolism resulting in ceramide and cholesterol ester accumulation in the ALS brain.

## 4.6 Inflammation and Neurodegeneration: Can We Measure Neuroprotection and Repair through Imaging Techniques?

Neurodegenerative diseases are mainly caused by a chronic or an acute exposure of the neurons to reactive oxygen intermediates (ROI) that may lead to cell suicide pathway (apoptosis) activated by the accumulation of toxic products of oxidative metabolism. The progression of these diseases can be slowed or halted using inorganic nanoparticles to scavenge ROI and thereby prevent the activation of apoptosis and the death of the cells. Recent findings have demonstrated that these specific nanoparticles can destroy ROI

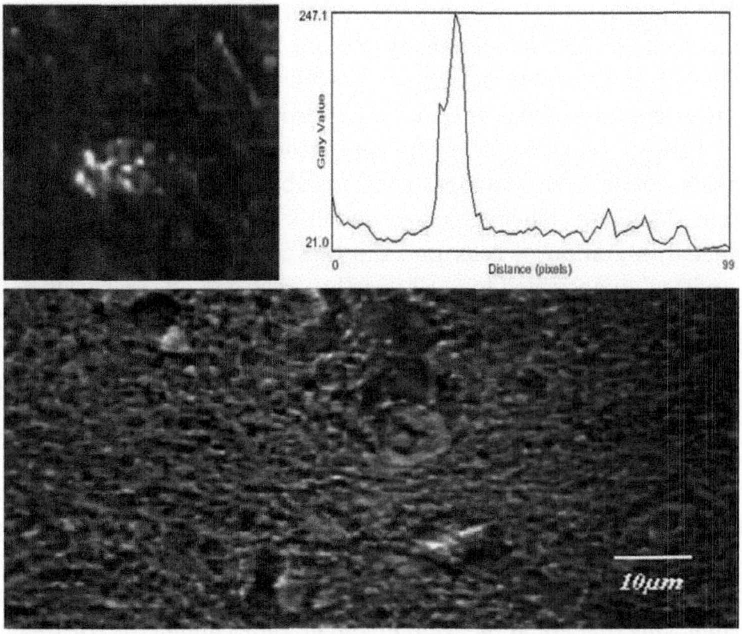


**Figure 4.9** SECARS image of CLUSPIO-treated ALS brain tissue, taken in the fingerprint region around 1660 $cm^{-1}$. The corresponding cross-section profile shows the intensity enhancement from the bright regions.

in retinal neurons in culture and can prevent ROI-mediated retinal degeneration in vivo.

Earlier studies on the evaluation of therapeutic efficacy for neurodegenerative diseases and neuroprotection through imaging techniques have showed that ultrasmall superparamagnetic particles of iron oxide (USPIO) may be a more specific MRI marker compared with gadolinium-DTPA (Gd). As such, use of USPIO-enhanced MRI provides more imaging information and reveals different enhancement patterns that may reflect the different stages of pathology. Research findings demonstrated that USPIO labeling of monocytes (using T1-weighted spin-echo, dual-echo T2-weighted spin-echo, and T2 gradient-echo (T2*)) appeared to be successful in vitro as well as in vivo for relapsing-remitting multiple sclerosis (MS) patients (Siemens Vision, Erlangen, Germany), screened monthly at 1.5 T. The predominant compartmentalization of USPIO into phagocytes or low concentrations of USPIO in vivo may justify the lack of T2* hypointensity. Recent studies have introduced SECARS microscopy as another enhanced imaging approach for early diagnosis of neurodegenerative disorders.

Several magnetic labeling approaches have been developed using coated SPIO nanoparticles to label stem and mammalian cells. Magnetic labeling allows monitoring of the temporal and spatial migration of cells into the CNS across the BBB. Research studies demonstrated that cells can be safely and effectively labeled using ferumoxides (SPIO nanoparticles approved by the United States Food and Drug Administration (FDA)), in combination with cationic transfection agents (e.g., poly-L-lysine) or FDA-approved agents (e.g., protamine sulfate). In therapeutic applications such as stroke or treatment of CNS tumors, labeled cells (i.e., embryonic, mesenchymal, hematopoietic, and neural stem cells) migrating toward areas of cerebral infarction or tumors can be monitored with cellular MR imaging.

MRI detection of SPIO-labeled cells may allow the evaluation of stem cells that could be used for repair, replacement, or treatment of CNS diseases. However, MR imaging cannot, as yet, determine the functional status and differentiation of magnetically labeled stem cells into neuronal cells. In clinical trials on spinal cord trauma models, magnetic cell labeling was still unable to distinguish hemorrhage and migration of labeled cells into areas of damage. This justifies the need to develop a multi-technique imaging approach to monitor cellular therapies.

A microemulsion methodology is implemented for developing novel biocompatible stealth nanoparticles for encapsulating drugs for brain delivery and optimizing BBB circumvention. Clinical trials showed that the presence of the stealth nanoparticles in the neurovasculature lacked significant effect on cerebral perfusion flow in vivo. Data (in vitro/vivo) also showed that the formulations had no significant effect on barrier integrity, membrane permeability, or alteration of expression of the BBB tight-junction proteins, occludin, and claudin-1. The implementation of in situ brain perfusion technique showed that uptake of the stealth nanoparticles across the BBB was significant and comparable to other neuropharmaceutical agents (e.g., caffeine, theophylline). Studies on electron microscopy demonstrated that nanoparticles remained intact after penetrating the brain extracellular space from the neurovasculature. The technology was also applied to increase the distribution of paclitaxel in the brain. This chemotherapeutic agent is active in various brain metastases in vitro but appears limited in actual efficacy because of p-glycoprotein-mediated brain efflux. Encapsulation of paclitaxel significantly increased brain drug uptake and increased toxicity toward p-glycoprotein-expressing tumor cells. Research findings showed that incorporation into stealth nanoparticles effectively masked the characteristics of paclitaxel that interact with p-glycoprotein.

## 4.7 Constraints in the Treatment of Neurodegenerative Diseases: Future Directions

The major problem with motor neuron disease is its diagnosis. Even though magnetic resonance imaging, positron emission tomography, single-positron emission computerized tomography, spinal fluid biochemistry, and other laboratory tests are helpful to identify and study the disease progression, a simple and effective diagnostic test is required to identify the disease at an early stage (mild cognitive impairment) of progression. Lack of awareness results in low rates of recognition of the disease by family members and physicians. In this context, a drug must cross the BBB to exhibit therapeutic activity. The homeostatic defense mechanism of the BBB strictly restricts the entry of many chemical substances, including drugs. Recent studies indicate that ALS pathology involves more complicated mechanisms; therefore, it is not so easy to develop a new drug that restricts all the complicated pathways involved in the development of neurodegenerative diseases.

Some neurodegenerative diseases have been found to be a multifactorial diseases with several pathogenetic mechanisms and pathways, which are not necessarily interrelated. Therefore, it would be a great step forward for ALS therapy if a multifunctional nanotechnology approach could be developed for designing therapeutic cocktails that simultaneously and specifically target the main molecular culprits involved in neurodegenerative diseases. Nevertheless, there are still many challenges regarding the biocompatibility of nanoparticles and nanodevices, especially in a complex biological milieu like the brain with a huge concentration of cells. Therefore, it seems that a long and puzzling path is ahead to make the envisioned nanoneurosurgical approaches of curing CNS diseases a practical technology and eventually a routine clinical practice.

In summary, tremendous efforts in the last several decades have resulted in numerous inventions to improve CNS drug delivery. Many of the systems have significant potential for clinical applications. Nonetheless, the wide variety of strategies signals the inherent difficulty in therapeutic and imaging agent transport across the BBB. In fact, the effective combination of several approaches, such as encapsulation of drugs into nanoparticles conjugated with vector moieties or using micelles of Pluronic block copolymers along with Pluronic unimers for drug efflux transporter inhibition in brain capillaries, may yield promising outcomes. With regard to the nervous system, studies of cell and molecular imaging are rapidly converging with the emerging impact of nanotechnology on CNS imaging and therapy. Although currently PET imaging agents appear to be more biochemically specific (i.e., FDG-PET), high-field MR imaging, surface-enhanced nanoimaging (SECARS) microscopy, and other novel nanodignostic techniques were clearly shown to have already impacted preclinical and clinical CNS imaging.

For instance, one form of iron oxide nanoparticle (ferumoxtran-10 USPIO) given intravascularly can target phagocytic cells (macrophages and astrocytes) in both neoplastic and nonneoplastic CNS lesions in both animal models and patients. Another type of iron oxide nanoparticle (ferumoxide SPIO) can be used in combination with protamine sulphate to label mononuclear white blood cells and stem cells. Such novel cellular contrast agents labeled with inert nanoparticles can enable visualization by MR imaging in vivo of as few as 100 lymphocytes trafficking to mouse spinal cord experimental allergic encephalitis lesions. Similarly SPIO-labeled stem cells can be imaged to be differentiated into endothelial cells vascularizing a glioma in vivo. Indeed, the initial clinical trials of cellular contrast agents using SPIO visualized on MR imaging have been demonstrated. In addition to the surface-enhanced properties of nanoparticles, their size and magnetic moment can be modulated depending on biological requirements. Nanoparticles can be conjugated to targeting agents such as chlorotoxin to specifically bind glioma cells. Stealth nanoparticles can ferry drugs or imaging agents across the BBB; these nanoparticles are normally substrates for endothelial efflux pathways (i.e., p-glycoprotein) and thereby excluded from the CNS. Indeed, even self-assembling high-epitope-attenuation nanofiber technology was reported to selectively guide differentiation of neural progenitor cells and to have impact in vivo on spinal cord injury; therefore, biotechnology is active in the merging areas of CNS imaging and nanomedicine.

Recently, the ability to package a variety of drugs in cells to affect neuroregeneration, curb anti-inflammatory activities, or prevent microbial infections within the CNS has received significant attention. All together these works lay an important foundation for future studies into improving pharmacokinetics, reducing system drug toxicity, and enabling earlier diagnosis of neurodegenerative disorders. It can be concluded that nanomedicines definitely sweep away the barriers of traditional drug targeting. Hence, it is beyond doubt that nanomedicine, especially when combined with tissue engineering and stem cell research, could provide new opportunities to change the method of diagnosis and treatment of ALS disease and improve the lifestyle of patients. Although this is a larger challenge, the ray of optimism coupled with knowledge will best show better results in the future.

## Further Reading

1. Gervasi NM, Kwok JC, Fawcett JW. Role of extracellular factors in axon regeneration in CNS. *Regener Med.* 2008;3:907–923.
2. McLachlan DR, Kruck TP, Lukiw WJ, Krishnan SS. Would decreased aluminum ingestion reduce the incidence of Alzheimer's disease. *CMAJ.* 1991;145:793–804.
3. Weissig V, Boddapati SV, Cheng S-M, D'Souza GGM. Liposomes and liposome-like vesicles for drug and DNA delivery to mitochondria. *J Liposome Res.* 2006;16:249–264.
4. Nazem A, Mansoori G. Nanotechnology for Alzheimer's disease: detection and treatment. *Insciences J.* 2011;1:169–193.

5. Pardridge W. The blood–brain barrier: bottleneck in brain drug development. *NeuroRx*. 2005;2:3–14.
6. Kingsley JD, Dou H, Morehead J, Rabinow B, Gendelman HE, Destache CJ. Nanotechnology: a focus on nanoparticles as a drug delivery system. *J Neuroimmunol Pharmacol*. 2006;1:340–350.
7. Kabanov AV, Batrakova EV. New technologies for drug delivery across the blood brain barrier. *Curr Pharm Des*. 2004;10:1355–1363.
8. Spector R. Drug transport in the mammalian central nervous system: multiple complex systems. A critical analysis and commentary. *Pharmacology*. 2000;60:58–73.
9. Alyaudtin R, Reichel A, Löbenberg R, Ramge P, Kreuter J, Begley DJ. Interaction of poly(butylcyanoacrylate) nanoparticles with the blood–brain barrier in vivo and in vitro. *J Drug Target*. 2001;9:209–221.
10. Pardridge W. Targeting neurotherapeutic agents through the blood–brain barrier. *Arch Neurol*. 2002;59:35–40.
11. Cornford EM, Cornford ME. New systems for delivery of drugs to the brain in neurological disease. *Lancet Neurol*. 2002;1:306–315.
12. Pardridge W. Drug and gene delivery to the brain: the vascular route. *Neuron*. 2002;36:555–558.
13. Misra A, Ganesh S, Shahiwala A, Shah SP. Drug delivery to the central nervous system: a review. *J Pharm Pharm Sci*. 2003;6:252–273.
14. Begley DJ. Delivery of therapeutic agents to the central nervous system: the problems and the possibilities. *Pharmacol Ther*. 2004;104:29–45.
15. Kas HS. Drug delivery to brain by microparticulate systems. *Adv Exp Med Biol*. 2004;553:221–230.
16. Banks W, Lebel C. Strategies for the delivery of leptin to the CNS. *J Drug Target*. 2002;10:297–308.
17. Loscher W, Potschka H. Drug resistance in brain diseases and the role of drug efflux transporters. *Nat Rev Neurosci*. 2005;6:591–602.
18. Liu X, Chen C. Strategies to optimize brain penetration in drug discovery. *Curr Opin Drug Discovery Dev*. 2005;8:505–512.
19. Mayhan W. Regulation of blood–brain barrier permeability. *Microcirculation*. 2001;8:89–104.
20. Smith MW, Gumbleton M. Endocytosis at the blood–brain barrier: from basic understanding to drug delivery strategies. *J Drug Target*. 2006;14:191–214.
21. Begley D. The blood–brain barrier: principles for targeting peptides and drugs to the central nervous system. *J Pharm Pharmacol*. 1996;48:136–146.

22. Tamai I, Tsuji A. Transporter-mediated permeation of drugs across the blood–brain barrier. *J Pharm Sci.* 2000;89:1371–1388.
23. Fromm M. P-glycoprotein: a defense mechanism limiting oral bioavailability and CNS accumulation of drugs. *Int J Clin Pharmacol Ther.* 2000;38:69–74.
24. Gaillard PJ, Visser CC, de Boer AG. Targeted delivery across the blood–brain barrier. *Expert Opin Drug Deliv.* 2005;2:299–309.
25. Liu G, Garrett MR, Men P, Zhu X, Perry G, Smith MA. Nanoparticle and other metal chelation therapeutics in Alzheimer disease. *Biochim Biophys Acta.* 2005;1741:246–252.
26. Garcia-Garcia E, Andrieux K, Gil S, Couvreur P. Colloidal carriers and blood–brain barrier (BBB) translocation: a way to deliver drugs to the brain. *Int J Pharm* 2005;298:274–292.
27. Silva GA. Neuroscience nanotechnology: progress, opportunities and challenges. *Nat Rev Neurosci.* 2006;7:65–74.
28. Zoccolella S, Beghi E, Palagano G, et al. Signs and symptoms at diagnosis of amyotrophic lateral sclerosis: a population-based study in southern Italy. *Eur J Neurol.* 2006;13:789–792.
29. Qureshi MM, Hayden D, Urbinelli L, et al. Analysis of factors that modify susceptibility and rate of progression in amyotrophic lateral sclerosis (ALS). *Amyotroph Lateral Scler.* 2006;7:173–182.
30. Shaw PJ. Molecular and cellular pathways of neurodegeneration in motor neurone disease. *J Neurol Neurosurg Psychiatr.* 2005;76:1046–1057.
31. Kadiu I, Glanzer JG, Kipnis J, Gendelman HE, Thomas MP. Mononuclear phagocytes in the pathogenesis of neurodegenerative diseases. *Neurotox Res.* 2005;8:25–50.
32. Watson G, Bastacky J, Belichenko P, et al. Intrathecal administration of AAV vectors for the treatment of lysosomal storage in the brains of MPS I mice. *Gene Ther.* 2006;13:917–925.
33. Minn A, Ghersi-Egea JF, Perrin R, Leininger B, Siest G. Drug metabolizing enzymes in the brain and cerebral microvessels. *Brain Res Brain Res Rev.* 1991;16:65–82.
34. Abbott N, Romero I. Transporting therapeutics across the blood–brain barrier. *Mol Med Today.* 1996;2:106–113.
35. Davson H, Segal MB. Physiology of the CSF and blood-brain barriers. In: *Special Aspects of the Blood–Brain Barrier.* Boca Raton: CRC Press; 1996:303–485.

36. Banks WA, Kastin AJ. Passage of peptides across the blood–brain barrier: pathophysiological perspectives. *Life Sci.* 1996;59: 1923–1943.
37. Langer R. Drug delivery. Drugs on target. *Science.* 2001;293:58–59.
38. Richards Grayson AC, Choi IS, Tyler BM, et al. Multi-pulse drug delivery from a resorbable polymeric microchip device. *Nat Mater.* 2003;2:767–772.
39. Andjus P, Bataveljic D, Vanhoutte G, et al. In vivo morphological changes in animal models of amyotrophic lateral sclerosis and Alzheimer's-like disease. *Anat Rec.* 2009;292:1882–1892.
40. Machtoub L, Bataveljic D, Andjus PR. Molecular imaging of brain lipid environment of lymphocytes in amyotrophic lateral sclerosis using magnetic resonance imaging and SECARS microscopy. *Physiol Res.* 2011;60(suppl 1):S121–S127.
41. Machtoub LH. Investigating neurodegenerative disorder systems using USPIO-nanoparticles with (SECARS) microscopy. *J Neurol.* 2010;257: S65–S68.
42. Machtoub LH. Monitoring the inflammatory process by surface enhanced nanoimaging microscopy. *Curr Neurovasc Res.* 2012;9(3):214–222.
43. Siepmann J, Siepmann F, Florence AT. Local controlled drug delivery to the brain: mathematical modeling of the underlying mass transport mechanisms. *Int J Pharm.* 2006;314:101–119.
44. Duncan R. The dawning era of polymer therapeutics. *Nat Rev Drug Discov.* 2003;2:347–360.
45. Gabizon A, Shmeeda H, Barenholz Y. Pharmacokinetics of pegylated liposomal doxorubicin: review of animal and human studies. *Clin Pharmacokinet.* 2003;42:419–436.
46. Feng SS, Mu L, Win KY, Huang G. Nanoparticles of biodegradable polymers for clinical administration of paclitaxel. *Curr Med Chem.* 2004;11:413–424.
47. Liu G, Garrett MR, Men P, Zhu X, Perry G, Smith MA. Nanoparticle and other metal chelation therapeutics in Alzheimer disease. *Biochim Biophys Acta.* 2005;1741(3):246–252.
48. Aebischer P, Schluep P, Deglon N, et al. Intrathecal delivery of CNTF using encapsulated genetically modified xenogeneetic cells in ALS patients. *Nat Med.* 1996;2:696–699.
49. Azzouz M. Gene therapy for ALS: progress and prospects. *Biochim Biophys Acta Mol Basis Dis.* 2006;1761:1122–1127.

50. Boisselier E, Astruc D. Gold nanoparticles in nanomedicine: preparations, imaging, diagnostics, therapies and toxicity. *Chem Soc Rev.* 2009;38:1759–1782.

51. Ekegren T, Hanrieder J, Bergquist J. Clinical perspectives of high-resolution mass spectrometry-based proteomics in neuroscience: exemplified in amyotrophic lateral sclerosis biomarker discovery research. *J Mass Spectrom.* 2008;43(5):559–557.

52. Nabeshi H, Yoshikawa T, Matsuyama K, et al. Systematic distribution, nuclear entry and cytotoxicity of amorphous nanosilica following topical application. *Biomaterials.* 2011;32:2713–2724.

# Chapter 5

# Novel Therapeutic Approaches

Treatments for ALS are divided into pharmacological (medicine), behavioral (physical therapy), and supportive, which is not designed to treat the disease but to prevent its complications. Currently, ALS has no cure; the conventional treatments are meant to slow its progression. ALS cannot be prevented, just as it cannot be cured. The small proportion of hereditary cases can be avoided by testing the fetus of parents who carry the genes that predict a high probability of ALS. Recent studies have shown promising therapeutic approaches based on cell replacement and gene therapy, which reflect current optimism as a viable strategy for the treatment of ALS and other neurodegenerative diseases.

## 5.1 Conventional Treatments for ALS

In its early stages, ALS usually goes unnoticed. This is particularly true for sporadic cases. This is so because the signs are not specific for ALS, and may not, at the start, be particularly troublesome. Once the diagnosis is made, the disease progresses over the next 3 to 5 years. During this progression, muscle strength is lost throughout

*Amyotrophic Lateral Sclerosis: Advances and Perspectives of Neuronanomedicine*
Lina Machtoub and Yu Kasugai

ISBN 978-981-4463-04-1 (Hardcover), 978-981-4463-05-8 (eBook)
www.panstanford.com

the body. Initially, mobility becomes a problem and patients become wheelchair- and bed-bound. They become incontinent (unable to control the bladder) and may be unable to self-feed. Usually the breathing muscles are the last to be affected. Once this happens, pneumonia and death result. The speed at which ALS progresses is variable. Progression and lifespan cannot be predicted. Those whose speech and swallowing are affected early have the worst outlook. Most people with ALS live three to 5 years. About 30% of patients with ALS live 5 years after diagnosis, and about 10%–20% live for more than 10 years. Riluzole (Rilutek) is the first and only medicine approved so far to delay the progression of ALS (Fig. 5.1). It sometimes delays the need for devices that assist breathing, such as a ventilator. It blocks several types of protein channels in the brain that allow calcium to enter neurons, including the N-methyl-D-aspartate (NMDA) receptor. Normally the NMDA receptor is activated by the amino acid glutamate. Over-activation of the receptor, and the massive influx of calcium, may contribute to the degeneration and death of motor neurons seen in ALS. In addition to the medication, the conventional treatments include speech and behavioral therapy, which can slow the progression of ALS and prevent aspiration pneumonia, often the cause of death in people with ALS. Physical therapy can be helpful in performing a range of motion activities and exercises to maintain strength and flexibility. Therapists can also assist with the use of a wheelchair and other devices (walker, braces, and ramps) that help with mobility.

## 5.2 Occupational Therapy and Supportive Therapy

Occupational therapists work with patients to maximize their achievement, competence, and satisfaction by improving both physical and psychological well-being. Examples of interventions may include assessment for electronic assistive technology such as environmental controls, housing adaptations, and help with eating and drinking. Drooling is a problem in people with ALS. Atropine is used to control drooling. Excessive saliva can also make someone more likely to have aspiration pneumonia. Muscle jerks and cramps

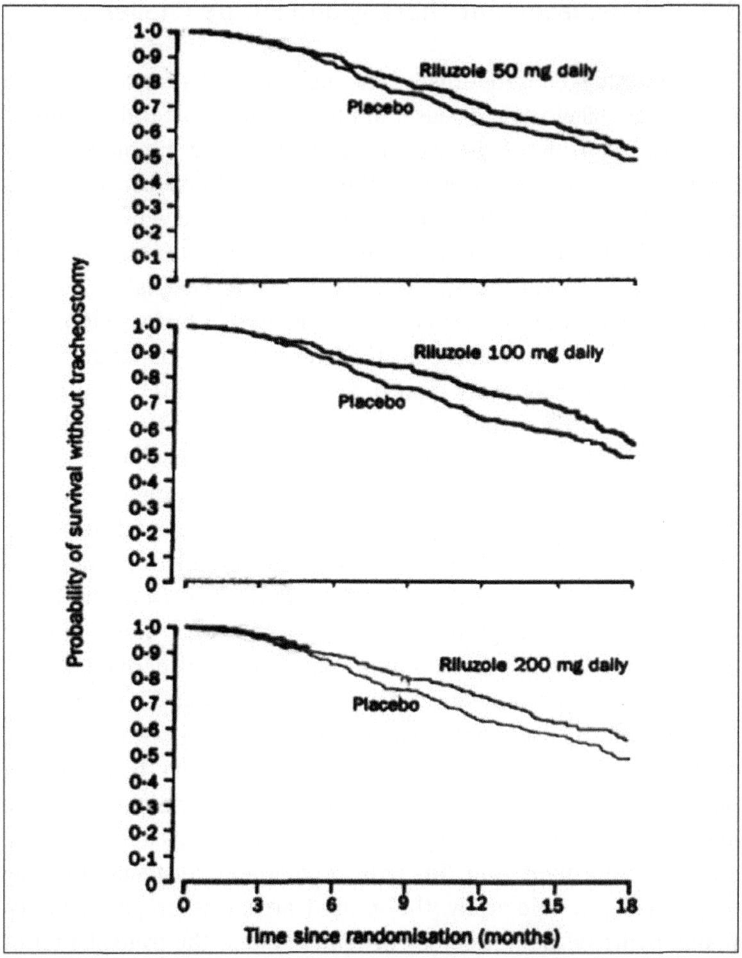


**Figure 5.1** Probability of survival without tracheostomy using the approved drug, riluzole.

in late-stage ALS can be reduced with muscle relaxants. In very advanced ALS, feeding may be impossible through the mouth, and feeding tubes may be needed. Eventually, when the breathing muscles are affected, patients need to have mechanically assisted ventilation.

## 5.3 Cell Replacement Therapy and Future Challenges

Serial neurodegenerative disorders, such as ALS, Parkinson's disease (PD), and Alzheimer's disease, induce extensive neural cell death. The treatment of the diseases requires not only inhibition of the progress but also recovery of the lost functions because these neural deaths are progressive. The condition in which specified neurons are lost in some particular brain area was quite suitable for cell replacement therapy. In 1979, the first two trials in rodents were reported. In those experiments, rats with 6-hydroxydopamine (6-OHDA)-induced lesions of the mesostriatal dopamine (DA) system unilaterally were transplanted rat fetal DA neurons. It was known already that rodents with those treatments exhibit a hemiparkinsonian-like syndrome with motor and cognitive deficits. The graft tissues were taken from the ventral mesencephalon of 13- to 15-day-old rat fetuses, and they were implanted directly into or adjacent to the 6-OHDA treatment striatum. The transplantation reduced the motor and cognitive deficits derived from the lesion protocol and the degree of behavioral recovery was found to be associated with the extent of the transplant-derived DA re-innervation of the previously denervated striatum. The recoveries were found in also nonhuman primates treated with N-methyl-4-phenyl-1,2,3,6-tetrahydropyridine (MPTP, which has selective neurotoxicity to dopaminergic neurons of the substantia nigra (SN) in human and in nonhuman primates), which persisted for 2 months after the transplantation. To confirm whether transplanted tissues functioned physiologically, the grafted area was prepared for tyrosine hydroxylase immunocytochemistry, and the transplantation experiments in rats showed synaptic contacts of both host-to-graft and graft-to-host present in the host brain. Moreover, the grafts exhibited spontaneously active action potential waveform and firing rates similar to those found in SN in situ. Quantification of transmitter metabolism and glucose utilization in the grafted area showed restoration of DA, and equivalent metabolic rates for the grafted tissue and the intact SN. The functional effects clearly come from the survival and continuous function of the graft. When the graft was removed or destroyed after transplantation, the deficits immediately reappeared.

Owing to these initial studies of fetal DA neurons in experimental Parkinsonism, the first clinical trials of transplantation were performed in PD, but with the patients' own adrenal medulla, not ventral mesencephalic tissue. Usage of human fetal tissue is linked to the ethical and immunological problems, to avoid them. Adrenal medulla cells were the alternative candidate of catecholamine-producing cells suitable for grafting (Fig. 5.2). Four patients with severe PD received adrenal medulla autotransplantation with stereotaxic procedure between 1982 and 1985. Two patients were grafted in the caudate neucleus and two in the putamen. There was no adverse effect in the transplantation, but minor improvements of motor function were observed for short term, from 2 to 6 months. Recent findings reported the first successful adrenal medulla autotransplantations in two young patients (35 and 39 years old) with PD. They used open microsurgical techniques and through the cerebral cortex implanted pieces of adrenal medulla cells into a premade cavity in the head of the caudate nucleus, instead of a stereotaxic procedure. Rigidity and akinesia had disappeared in the first patient at 10 months after surgery, and the second patient at 3 months, respectively. Because of the dramatic improvements, many similar operations were done to reproduce the results. For example, 19 of the patients with severe PD were followed for 6 months after adrenal medulla autotransplantation. The mean percentage of on time, the hours of the waking day when the antiparkisonian medications were effective, increased from 48% to 75% at 6 months after the surgery. The dosages of antiparkinsonian drugs could not be decreased after the operation. There were certainly some improvements in these surgeries, but it is a serious problem with this procedure that the mechanisms of improvement are largely unknown. It seems unlikely that the reduction of Parkinsonian symptoms is due to catecholamine release from the implanted cells as originally intended. Few cases of autopsy showed no surviving graft or very limited number of presumed adrenal medulla cells. Those reports suggest that survival of the graft is not necessary. Series of experiments with MPTP-treated mice or monkeys showed tyrosine hydroxylase-immunoreactive fibers after grafting adrenal medullary tissue into the brain, and the fibers appeared to be from the host, not the grafted. These studies suggest that the grafting

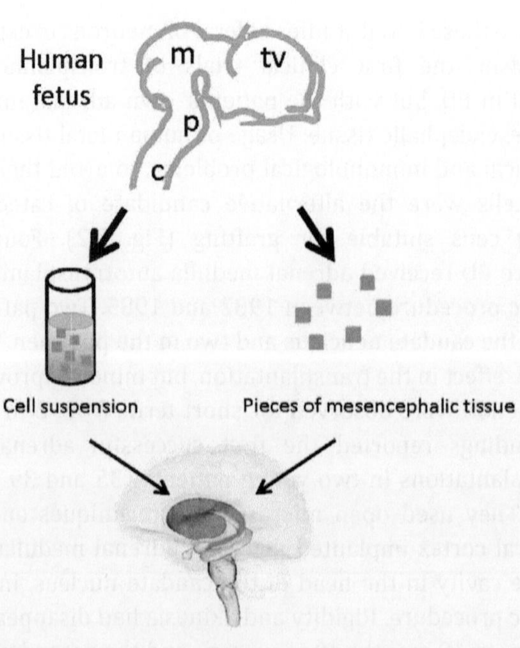


**Figure 5.2** Diagram of the transplantation therapy for Parkinson's disease. The ventral mesencephalon of human fetal DA neurons was prepared as a cell suspension, or divided in pieces into the caudate nucleus. tv = telencephalic vesicle, m = mesencephalic flexure, p = pontine flexure, c = cervical flexure.

of adrenal medullary cells or operational procedure stimulated a neurotorophic action and induced recovery of remaining host dopaminergic neurons. The first stage of this transplantation therapy got moving in the late 1980s, but disappeared rapidly in the 1990s.

Parallely, abilities of fetal SN were explored. In a series of experiments, human fetal DA neurons were implanted into the DA-denervated striatum of immunosuppressed rats. It was confirmed that transplanted human fetal DA neurons can survive in rodents and the optimal age of the donor was found to be 8 to 10 gestational weeks. The transplanted DA cells reinnervated the entire striatum of MPTP-treated rats and tyrosine hydroxylase immunoreactive terminal made asymmetric contacts with spines of the host animals. After confirmation of safety, intrastriatal grafts of human fetal DA neurons were transplanted into two 50-year-old women with severe PD. Immunosuppression (cyclosporine, azathioprine, and prednisolone) was given from 2 days before the transplantation, and ventral mesencephalic tissue from four fetuses was implanted stereotaxically on the side contralateral to that exhibiting the more severe symptoms. The same doses of levodopa were taken during the 6 months preceding the operation and the 6 months of postoperative period. As for results from up to 6 months postoperatively, there were some effects derived from the transplantations for these patients: (i) There was no striking change in the mean time spent "on" during the first 6 postoperative months. (ii) There was a small but significant improvement in the motor performance. (iii) The duration of the response to a single levodopa dose did not change significantly. (iv) The motor readiness potential increased gradually during off times. This potential is a slowly rising negative electroencephalographic potential, and elicited from 0.5 to 1.5 s before a voluntary movement. (v) Positron emission tomography (PET) did not show any increase of 6-L-[18F]-fluorodopa uptake in the grafted striatum. These results suggest that the transplantation of fetal DA neurons may have provided a modest improvement in motor function.

The method also showed a small improvement for the patients. Symptomatic relief was marked and sustained due to improvement of the transplantation technique and optimal condition to store transplanted tissues. In a reported study, the initial treatment for a patient, 49 years old, with L-dopa was successful, but he developed progressively worsening on–off phenomena after 7 years. At the operation, the duration and frequency of off periods were relatively stable and he had four to five daily off periods and spent 40% to 50% of the time in a severe off state on the average. PET scan showed the left putamen markedly deficient in DA-synthesizing capacity (the right side was also, but it was to a lesser extent). Dissociated ventral mesenchepalic tissue from four fetuses (8 to 9 weeks of age) was implanted in the anterior, middle, and posterior part of the left putamen. Surprisingly, both the time spent in the off period and the number of daily off periods were reduced dramatically during the 2 months after the operation. The rigidity in his right arm also progressively reduced. These progress persisted at least 5

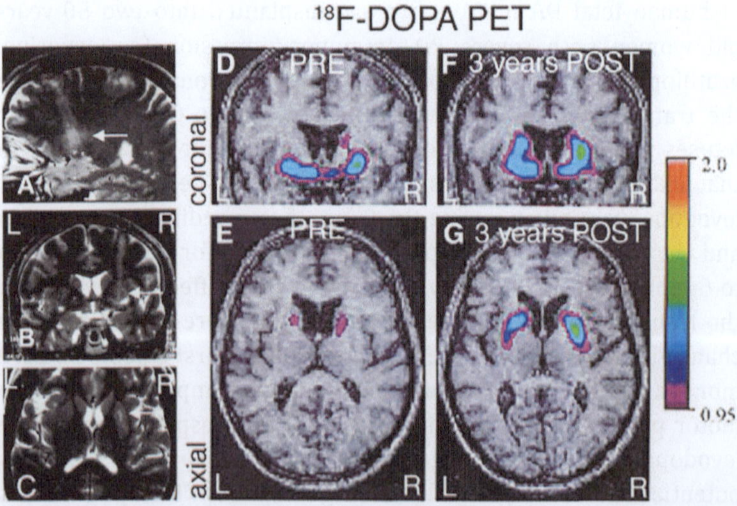


**Figure 5.3** (A–C) MRI study performed 24 hours after the first surgery (patient 1). The four parallel needle tracks through the right putamen are visible in the axial (C) and sagittal (A). (D–G) Parametric maps of F-DOPA uptake (Ki) overlaid on the patient's MRI. (D–E) A preoperative PET scan showed a marked, asymmetrical decrease in putaminal 18F-DOPA uptake in the first patient, consistent with the diagnosis of idiopathic Parkinson's disease. (F–G) Twenty-eight months after transplantation the PETs show a significant increase in 18F-DOPA uptake, more pronounced in the right putamen (>300% compared with preoperative values) than on the left (100% increase). R = right; L = left. Reproduced with permission from Mendez et al., *Brain*, 128, 1498–1510 (2005).

months after the transplantation. PET scan showed 30% increase of tracer uptake in the transplanted (left) putamen 5 months after the operation, when compared to that recorded 12 months before surgery. Though the uptake of 6-L-[18F] fluorodopa was lower in the left putamen than that of the right putamen before the operation (the ratio of left to right was 0.5), the ratio became 0.98 after the transplantation. Adding small refinements, this therapy improved to alleviate motor deficits in PD patients (Fig. 5.3, Tables 5.1 and 5.2).

In some cases, the patients with transplants could stop L-DOPA application completely. It was shown that the efficacy of this method was clearer in young patients than in older patients and it required new diagnosis to find the symptoms at an early stage.

**Table 5.1** (patient 1) Preoperative and last postoperative (3 years follow-up) UPDRS scores. PET studies indicated increase in 18F-DOPA uptake bilaterally. Reproduced with permission from Mendez et al., *Brain*, 128, 1498–1510 (2005)

**Table 1A** Functional outcome 3 years after transplantation: patient 1

| Measure | Baseline | 3 years after transplantation | Change |
|---|---|---|---|
| UPDRS | | | |
| Motor | | | |
| Off | 50 | 23 | 54% |
| On | 30 | 16 | 47% |
| Total | | | |
| Off | 97 | 67 | 31% |
| On | 78 | 58 | 25% |
| Dyskinesia scores | 12 | 8 | 34% |
| % time in Off | 50% | 25% | 50% |
| Pro/sup | | | |
| Right | | | |
| Off | 15 | 23 | 53% |
| On | 19 | 24 | 26% |
| Left | | | |
| Off | 14 | 23 | 64% |
| On | 15 | 22 | 47% |
| [$^{18}$F]fluorodopa $K_i$ | | | |
| Right putamen | 0.00174 | 0.007068 (28 months) | 306% |
| Left putamen | 0.003355 | 0.005205 (28 months) | 98% |

The recovery of motor function with grafted DA neurons is dependent on the survivability of the neurons, efficacy of innervation from the cells, and so on. To improve long-term survival of the grafted cells, it is the most important that the standardized protocol be established and improved to be optimistic, but it is quite hard. The protocols for the transplantation have been quite variable because they are dependent on how cells were obtained, prepared, preserved, and so forth. Unfortunately these points cannot be

**Table 5.2** (patient 2) Preoperative and last postoperative (3 years follow-up) UPDRS scores. PET studies indicated increase in 18F-DOPA uptake bilaterally. Reproduced with permission from Mendez et al., *Brain*, 128, 1498–1510 (2005)

**Table 1B** Functional outcome 3 years after transplantation: patient 2

| Measure | Baseline | 3 years after transplantation | Change |
|---|---|---|---|
| UPDRS | | | |
| Motor | | | |
| Off | 84 | 44 | 48% |
| On | 42 | 33 | 22% |
| Total | | | |
| Off | 155 | 84 | 46% |
| On | 102 | 73 | 28% |
| Dyskinesia scores | 23 | 2 | 91% |
| % time in Off | 50% | 25% | 50% |
| Pro/sup | | | |
| Right | | | |
| Off | 5 | 7 | 40% |
| On | 26 | 19 | –27% |
| Left | | | |
| Off | 8 | 23 | 187% |
| On | 22 | 22 | 0% |
| [$^{18}$F] fluorodopa $K_i$ | | | |
| Right putamen | 0.001578 | 0.005088 | 222% |
| Left putamen | 0.003493 | 0.001898 | –45% |
| Right midbrain | 0.001827 | 0.003474 | 90% |
| Left midbrain | 0.002467 | 0.003025 | 22% |

avoided from each situation, but some biochemical components and factors are investigated to improve the survivability of granted DA neurons. The compounds and methods are investigated to increase innervation from the grafted cells to transplanted striatum. For example, it is known that application of growth factor such as glial cell line-derived neurotrophic factor (GDNF) and substances can improve the survival of the neurons. This neurotrophic factor acts specifically on dopaminergic neurons and substantially increases the survival and differentiation of DA neurons in vitro and even in vivo. In recent studies, human ventral mesencephalic cells were stored in GDNF for 6 days at 4°C prior to the operation and implanted the cells bilaterally in postcommissural putamen of two patients. Preclinical studies showed that the mesencephalic cells stored with GDNF differentiated into tyrosine hydroxylase-positive cells, and the ratio was 1.4 times higher than that of the cells without GDNF. The pre- and postoperative scores for each patient significantly improved 15 months after follow-up. PET scanning indicated that the operation increased the uptake of 6-L-[18F]-fluorodopa by approximately 2 times. To improve the survivability of grafted cells, circumstances surrounding the grafted cell may be one of the critical factors involved in optimizing clinical outcomes.

The extent of reinnervation by grafted DA neurons in the striatum is related to the efficacy in the recovery of motor function. As complexity and accuracy in neural network is thought, it is reasonable that re-innervation and re-establishment of synaptic connection by the grafted cells to a specific subregion of the striatum helps the recovery of function. Some reports indicated that the distribution of DA neurons throughout the striatum using multiple injection site scan ensures that axonal coverage of the denervated area is optimized. In recent findings, neuroscientists compared the efficacy of a number of deposits in the survivability of grafted cells in animal models. The cells from the ventral mesencephalon of embryonic day 14 rat fetuses were transplanted into the head of the caudate-putamen of model rats, in a different way. One way was eighteen 0.2 μL deposits disseminated over six needle penetrations and the other was two 1.8 μL deposits centrally in the putamen. When the efficacies were compared 4 months after the operation, the eighteen-deposit method showed higher tyrosine hydroxylase immunohistochemistry to be 2.8-fold than that in the two-deposit method. Moreover, the outgrowth of graft-derived tyrosine hydroxylase-positive fiber was more extensive in the eighteen-deposit method. The results showed that distribution of the fetal nigral tissue in multiple small deposits provides for increased DA neurons survival. It is thought that the small-sized graft deposits increase contact between the implanted cells and the surrounding host striatal tissue. Sequential applications such as this experiment showed an increase in the efficacy in clinical studies.

Multiple transplantations improved multiple sites. The nigral grafts were basically placed in the ontogenic site, SN, but the results, particularly clinical outcomes, have not been enough to increase the quality of life in PD patients. Therefore, it is suggested that difficulty of the grafted cell grow their axons over long distances to reach their striatal target. The difficulty may be derived from no appropriate guidance cues in the mature host brains. Moreover, it has been demonstrated that simultaneous double grafts into both intrastriatum and intranigra might promote reconstruction of the nigrostriatal pathway and a better behavioral recovery in the rodent model of 6-OHDA-induced PD. It is known that DA is released in the substantia nigra (SN) pars reticulata by dendrites of pars compacta neurons. This dendritic release of DA activates D1 receptors expressed on the descending striatonigral axon terminals, and the D1 receptor activation inhibits striatonigral GABA release in the ventromedial thalamus to increase pars reticulata neuronal activity. The existence of the bidirectional pathway indicates a possibility that efferent nigrostriatal connections are not enough, but afferent striatonigral connections are also important to restore the function. Intranigral transplantation of fetal SN allografts showed behavioral recovery in rodents and primates. These animal experiments indicate that SN may be one of main targets for transplantation therapy. This "double graft" was operated in three patients with PD, and they were followed up for up to 13 months after the transplantations. Three patients with PD underwent bilateral transplantation of the fetal ventral mesencephalus into the putamen and SN. The surgical procedures were separated into two stages 4 weeks apart, and one side of the patients' brain received the operation in each stage. Interestingly, the double graft method was combined with GDNF application to store the fetal cells and multi-deposits (Fig. 5.4).

One of the patients had a hypertensive hemorrhage in the right frontal lobe 3 months after the transplantation, and the patient was followed for 3 months. The hemorrhage was confined to the subcortical white matter and did not reach the putamen, and it was thought that the hemorrhage was not due to the operation itself. Without

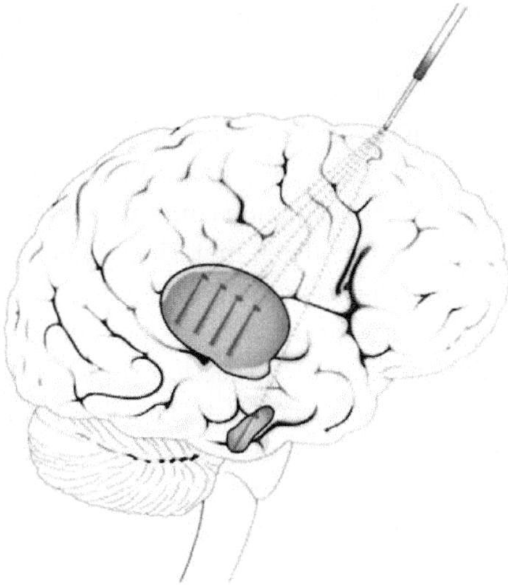

**Figure 5.4** Diagram illustrating the double transplant strategy. Four graft deposits are implanted into the putamen and one is implanted into the SN. Reproduced with permission from Mendez et al., *J. Neurosurg.*, 96, 589–596 (2002).

it, there were no intraoperative or perioperative complications. As a result, the operation showed obvious improvements in clinical outcome. The timed motor task of hand pronation/supination scores also improved bilaterally. Moreover, one of the three patients did not have a decrease in levodopa requirement, but the others showed a decrease of about 50% in the requirement after the surgery. PET scans also indicated an increase in [18F] fluorodopa Ki values of all patients. This positive result indicates that an appropriate target for transplantation, which focuses on reinnervation for well-suited brain region to rebuild the neuronal network, is crucial for transplantation therapy.

The other challenge to overcome in this transplantation therapy is avoiding graft-induced dyskinesias. The effect of this therapy has been highly variable and it is apparent in dyskinesias induced with L-DOPA. The mechanism of the dyskinesias is not clear, but the differences in the preparation and storage of the fetal tissue before grafting are suggested as one of the reasons. The patients who received tissue that had been stored for 1–8 days developed more pronounced off-phase dyskinesia than patients implanted with fresh tissue. On the basis of recent studies, it is suggested that this large variability is derived from how to dissect or prepare the fetal tissue, and that differences in tissue dissection are likely to change the ratio in types of the cells in the graft cells. In this study it is proposed that the fetal ventral mesencephalon contains approximately 5% DA neurons and that there are also a majority of glial cells, serotonin, GABA encephalin, and substance P positive neurons in the grafted tissue as a mixed composition. The proportion of these cells is dependent on the method of dissection and the formulation of the graft, suspension, and pieces of tissue. The DA neurobrasts in the ventral mesencephalon are also not a homogeneous population but comprise two major subtypes, and they differentiate A9 DA neurons in the substantianigra pars compacta (SNpc)and A10 DA neurons in the ventral tegmental area (VTA). These neurons are different in morphology and expression of some proteins (Girk2, calbindin, and Raldh1). Moreover, A9 DA neurons give rise to the nigrostriatal pathway and A10 DA neurons innervate the mesolimbic and mesocortical pathways. Transplantation experiment of rodents indicated that Girk2-positive neurons in SNpc dominantly innervate the host dorsal striatum, whereas VTA neurons preferentially made projections into the frontal cortex. On the other hand, non-DA neurons of the grafted cells, particularly serotonin and GABA neurons, spread broadly and within suspended graft. It is thought that the dyskinesia is due to the multi-composition of the grafted cells with large variability of function and innervation. Carlsson and colleagues compared L-DOPA-induced dyskinesia with mixture of serotonin neurons and DA neurons to evaluate the effect of the serotonin neurons. The authors identified rhombencephalic isthmus and performed the caudal cut at 1–1.5 mm rostral to the isthmus, to yield about one-half of the midbrain. A dorsal cut was done through the midbrain to limit the tissue to the ventral third of the piece. In rat model experiments, both the transplanted DA and serotonin neurons survived well after grafting to the striatum. DA neuron-rich grafts showed a significant (about 60%) reduction of L-DOPA-induced dyskinesia. The effect sustained for at least more than 10 weeks after the transplantation. These reports suggest the proportion of DA neurons relative to other neuronal cell types, and

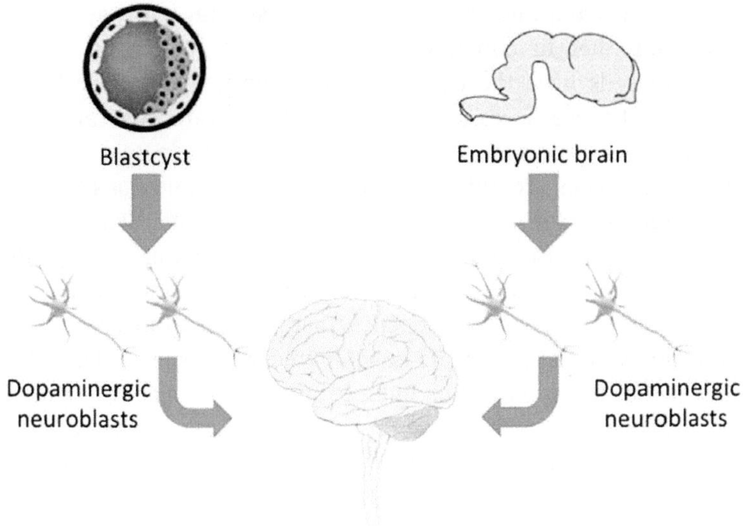


**Figure 5.5** Schematic illustration of different strategies to generate DA neurons for cell replacement in Parkinson's disease, starting from embryonic stem cells (left), from regionally specified progenitors, or committed DA neuron precursors in the embryonic brain (right).

their respective and appropriate innervations determine successful clinical outcome.

## 5.4 Stem Cell Transplantation Therapy

The clinical benefit from transplantation of ventral mesencephalic DA neurons seems to be improving gradually, although there are still some challenges to overcome in the therapy (Fig. 5.5). In recent findings, it has been shown that the grafted mesencephalic tissue had survived and kept the effects over 10 years, and that tissue or those cells could restore appropriate release of DA in the nigrostriatal system. To get more symptomatic relief in patients after the transplantation, one should focus on the functional aspects in detail. The grafted cells have to be functionally integrated into host basal ganglia-thalamo-cortical neural networks. With the integration, the appropriate afferent and efferent connections can be reconstructed and the impaired nigrostriatal pathway can be restored to their functional state.

Stem cells have the capacity to differentiate into all relevant neural cell types necessary to replace degenerated neural tissue. There are two ways to use the stem cell with pluripotent differentiation. The cells are differentiated in vitro to DA neurons prior to transplantation for the patient. This step could standardize the stem cells and control the quality in advance, particularly in regard to the purity of the cells. Moreover, stem cells can divide to self-renew and generate more committed progenies that give rise to specific tissues in the body, so the cells could be unlimited as the source. The other way is that the stem cell or induced progenitor cells differentiate into DA neurons in vivo after the transplantation, in the striatum and SN. There is a possibility that those differentiated neurons may integrate and reconstruct the nigrostriatal pathway better than the former way. In any case, one must know the mechanisms for the immature stem or progenitor cells to differentiate into the missing neuronal tissue. If this cell therapeutic approach can be available for the clinical stage, it will be next standard therapy for not only PD but also other neurodegenerative diseases such as ALS, Alzheimer's, and spinal cord injury.

Embryonic stem (ES) cell and human ES (hES) cell lines are derived from the cells of the inner cell mass of the blastocyst and are pluripotent. The specification can be controlled with the interplay of endogenous and exogenous factors. The ES cells can be differentiated into three distinct germ layers: the endoderm, the ectoderm, and the mesoderm. The cells committed to these germ layers grow to the cells of the tissues, including neurons and astrocytes. This feature of ES cells was appropriate for the regenerative therapy for neurodegenerative disorders. As a strategy, the ES cells are induced to specialized cells for therapies and cultured in dishes, and then they are transplanted into the patients. Specific functional neurons for neurodegenerative disorders can be generated from ES cells.

There are have been several studies to establish a method to generate specific neurons in high yield. In recent studies, sonic hedgehog, basic fibroblast growth factor 8, and ascorbic acid have been used to increase the yield of ES-derived thyrosine hydroxylase (TH)-positive neurons. Electrophysiological study showed that the neurons responded to direct application of GABA and glutamate, and spontaneous activity. In 2002, neuroscientists succeeded in differentiating ES cell lines of primates, cynomolgus monkeys, into DA neurons. These neurons released DA and extended neurites into the mouse striatum 2 weeks after the transplantation. hES cells were also tried as source of cells for applications in regenerative therapy. Previous findings reported directed differentiation of hES cells into tissue specific cells such as spinal motoneurons or midbrain DA neurons. The method for differentiation of the ES cells shows progressing steps in the laboratory level, but there are still some challenges to surmount. One of them is that there are considerable safety concerns for ES cells related to their potential for teratoma formation or neural overgrowth. The other is that DA neurons from hES cells could not show enough performance in vivo. Recent studies presented novel floor-plate-based strategy for the derivation of human DA neurons that efficiently engraft in vivo and yielded a significant, substantial, and long-lasting restitution of motor function. The studies were focused on the polarity of some transcription factors detectable during midbrain DA neuron development, such as LMX1A and FOXA2. The midbrain coexpresses the floor-plate (FP) marker FOXA2 and the roof-plate marker LMXA1 during the development. Usually floor-plate and roof-plate cells are located at distinct areas in the central nervous system and these cells migrate diametrically during the development (ventral or dorsal). There is a possibility that the gradient of these molecules or the downstream molecules decide the fate of precursors. This strategy induced more differentiation for DA neurons than conventional methods. A major challenge in the field has been the ability to generate functional DA neurons that engraft in vivo without the risk of neural overgrowth or inappropriate differentiation into non-midbrain neurons. It is thought that neural overgrowth is caused by primitive anterior neuroectodermal cell within the graft, and it is important whether the induced DA neurons are matured or not. When the DA neurons were transplanted into immunosuppressed mice for 4.5 months, the graft cores were defined with TH and human-specific NCAM and overgrowth was not detected. Rat models of PD grafted with DA neurons showed improvements in the stepping test, measuring forelimb akinesia, and in the cylinder test, assays that do not depend on pharmacological stimulation of the DA system. Moreover, grafting studies in adult MPTP-lesioned rhesus monkeys demonstrated robust DA neurons survival 1 month after the transplantation. Those graft cores were surrounded by TH-positive fibers. These results indicate that appropriate induction for ES cells into the specific cells support survival and function of the cells and suppress unanticipated overgrowth and teratoma formation. The growth and functions of hES-derived cells were compared with different stages of neural differentiation implanted in the brains of monkey models. The hES cells were matured by culture for 42 days with BDNF (brain-derived neurotrophic factor) and GDNF (glial cell line-derived neurotorophic factor) treatment. The matured and grafted hES cells survived in the brain of the monkeys as primarily dopaminergic neurons without tumorigenicity. On the other hand, undifferentiated ES cells expressing ES cell markers induced tumor formation in the monkey brain. The monkeys with the matured cells showed behavioral improvement for at least 12 months. This result supports effective validity of regenerative therapy with hES cells.

## 5.5 Clinical Applications of Cell Transplant Therapy

The first clinical experience of patients treated with cells derived from hES cells was done by Steven Schwartz and colleagues. A patient with Stargardt macular dystrophy (the most common pediatric macular degeneration) and a patient with dry age-related macular degeneration (ARMD) received a subretinal injection of hES cell-derived retinal pigment epithelium (RPE). Both disorders are associated with degeneration of the RPE, which induces loss of photoreceptor and progressive vision deficiency. The hES cells were differentiated into RPE in culture with over 99% ratio. In a preclinical study to test tumorigenicity and biodistribution, the hES cell-derived RPE was injected subretinally into immunosuppressed mice. There were no adverse effects or safety issues in any animals, and the differentiated hRPE cells survived for the lifetime (about 9 months) of the mice. Without immunostatining for the hRPE cells, the cells looked to be integrated into the mouse RPE layer (Fig. 5.6).

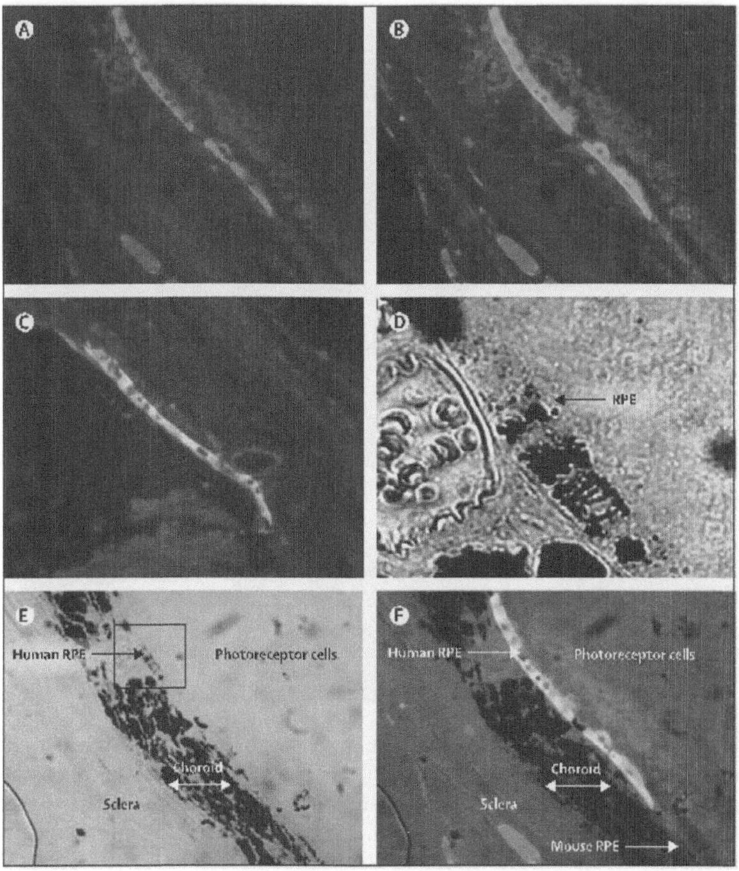


**Figure 5.6** Survival and integration of RPE generated from hESC-MA09 into an NIH III mouse eye after 9 months. Section stained with antihuman mitochondria (A) and antihuman bestrophin (B). Note the precise colocalization of human mitochondria and bestrophin staining in the same cells (C: A and B merged) and absence of staining in mouse RPE (F: A, B, C, and E merged). Frame on the bright field image (E) is enlarged in D to show morphology of human RPE. Magnification ×200 (A–C, E, and F); D is additionally magnified ×4–5. RPE = retinal pigment epithelium, hESC = human embryonic stem cells, NIH = National Institutes of Health. Reproduced with permission from Scwarltz et al., *Lancet*, 379, 713–720 (2012).

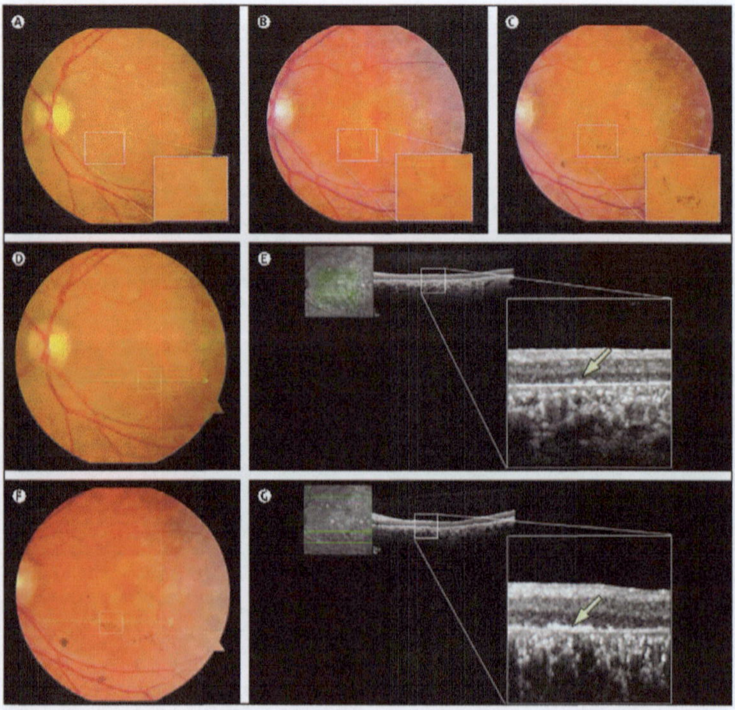

**Figure 5.7** Images of the hESC-RPE transplantation site in the patient with Stargardt macular dystrophy. Color fundus photographs of the patient's left macula preoperatively and postoperatively (A–C). The region inside the rectangle bisects the border of the surgical transplantation site and corresponds to macular atrophy not included in the surgical injection. (A) Baseline macular color image with widespread RPE and neurosensory macular atrophy. (B) Color macular image 1 week after hESC-RPE transplantation. Note the mild pigmentation most evident in the region of baseline RPE atrophy. This pigmentation increased at week 6 (C). (D–G) Color fundus photographs and SD-OCT images at baseline (D) and month 3 after transplant (F). Color images show increasing pigmentation at the level of the RPE from baseline to month 3. Registered SD-OCT images (E, G) show that increasing pigmentation is at the level of the RPE, normal monolayer RPE engraftment, and survival at month 3 (arrow) adjacent to region of bare Bruch's membrane devoid of native RPE. Reproduced with permission from Scwarltz et al., *Lancet* 379, 713–720 (2012).

50,000 induced retinal epithelium cells were injected into the subretinal space of one eye in each patient. There was no significant hyperproliferation, abnormal growth, or immune-mediated transplant rejection in either patient during the first 4 months. Color fundus photographs and SD-OCT (spectral domain ocular coherence tomography) image showed that transplanted hES cell-RPE survived and engrafted in the patient with Stargardt macular dystrophy (Fig. 5.7).

Particularly, SD-OCT indicated that the transplanted cells seem to have involved regions of complete pretransplant RPE loss as well as regions of pretransplant RPE compromise. Interestingly, both patients indicated functional visual improvements. At baseline, the central vision of the patient with Stargardt macular dystrophy was hand motions only, but best corrected visual acuity improved to counting fingers and seeing only one letter in the eye chart by 2 weeks, and to a stable level of five letters after 4 weeks. The patient also had subjective improvement in color vision, contrast, and dark adaptation in the treated eye. These results suggest effective possibility of ES cell therapy in humans.

## 5.6 Trials of Other Cell Sources for Stem Cell Therapy

As indicated above, biosafety and efficacy in stem cell therapy are dependent on how to control the differentiation, how the cells are matured, and how to secure enough number of the cells. There are some different sources of stem cells under investigation, including neural stem cells in embryonic brain, neural stem cells in adult brain, stem cells in other tissues, and so on (Fig. 5.8).

Controlled conversion of neuroepithelial precursors into DA neurons was first reported in 1998. Cells from ventral mesencephalon of the embryo were dissociated and cultured in medium supplemented with basic fibroblast growth factor (bFGF). Upon removal of the mitogen, approximately 20% of the total cell population was immunoreactive for TH. The expanded cells were transplanted into the ipsilateral striatum of adult rats treated with 6-OHDA. Those animals could moderately alleviate behavioral deficits 80 days after transplantation. In other studies dopaminergic

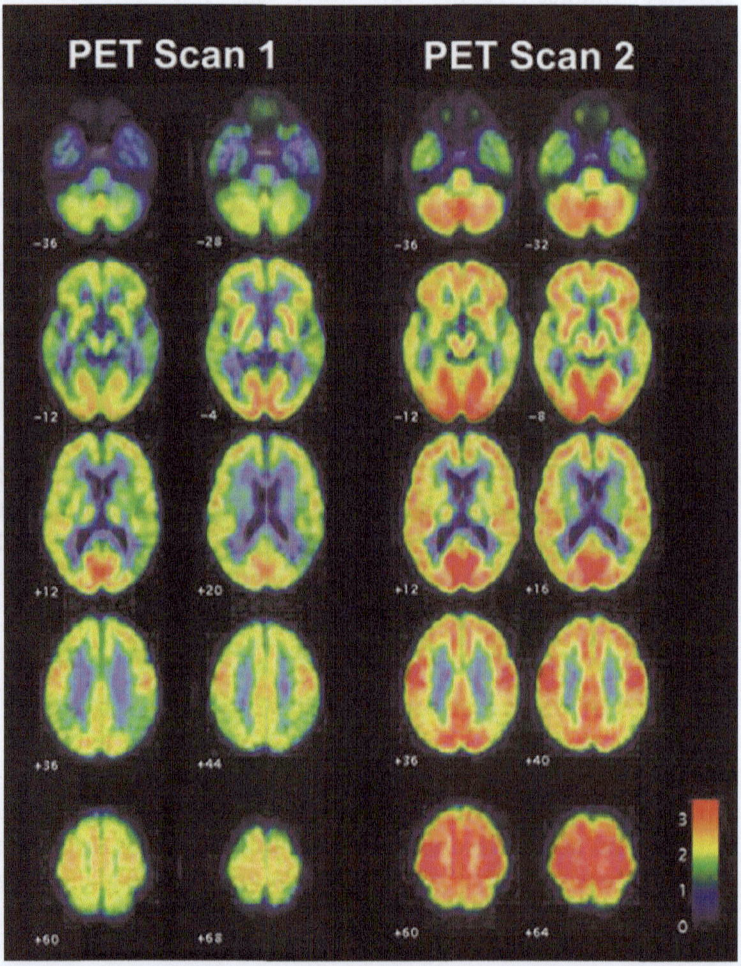


**Figure 5.8** PET scans. Averaged FDG PET scans in four subjects treated with NGF, overlaid on standardized MRI templates. Representative axial sections, with 6–8 months between first and second scan, showing widespread interval increases in brain metabolism. Flame scale indicates FDG use/100 g tissue/min; red color indicates more FDG use than blue. Reproduced with permission from Tuszynski et al., *Nat. Med.*, 11, 551–555 (2005).

phenotype was induced in an immortalized multipotent mouse stem cell line with overexpression of Nurr-1. Nurr-1 directly is crucial for TH expression and the mutations are associated with PD and schizophrenia.

For the introduction of neural stem cells into a certain fate, soluble extrinsic factors and essential intrinsic factors such as transcription factors are necessary. In the case of the generation of DA neurons, transcription factors including Nurr-1, NgN2, FoxA2, and other factors were transduced or transfected to the neural stem cells.

Neural stem cells were also found in adult animal and human brains. Recently, neuroscientists produced TH-expressing cells from the adult mouse subependyma of the lateral ventricle in vitro. The induction was done in FGF2 and glial cell-conditioned media. It has been found that neuronal replacement occurred after injury in the adult brain of stroke model. Moreover, for short-term growth factors FGF-2 (fibroblast growth factor 2) and EGF (epidermal growth factor), treatment stimulated not only the proliferation of endogenous progenitors but also their differentiation into neurons. Some recent studies reported population of progenitor cells in the SNpc of the adult brain. Those cells differentiate into glial cells in situ but not to neurons. However, when the freshly isolated progenitor cells are transplanted into the hippocampus, these cells can give rise to neurons. These results indicate that progenitor cells reside in the adult brain and they can differentiate into new neurons under the appropriate environmental signals.

These findings indicate the possibility that the patient's own neural stem cells could be available for generation of specific neurons. The advantage of this possibility could be the lack of any immune reaction. However, some problems can be expected. The source of neural stem cells is located in the deep area of the brain and its inaccessibility makes it more difficult in clinical utility. Multiple operations must also strain the patients. The other problem is that these cells might be impaired by age, the disease itself, and medical treatment.

To avoid these problems, there are many trials to find other sources of neural stem cells. These days, non-central nervous system-derived somatic multipotent stem cells are being focused on, to be less invasive. For instance, bone marrow stromal cells, mesenchymal stem cells derived from bone marrow cells, human dermis, human pulp tissue, and so on can be successfully induced into multipotent stem cells. To date, five types of dental tissue derived progenitor cell populations were identified, and it suggests the possibility that mesenchymal stem cells in specific tissues have led to the discovery of a variety of stem cells in every organ and tissue in the body. However, the precise features among these different multipotent stem cells remain unclear. For example, it is suggested that the neurogenicity of dental stem cells may be more potent than that of multipotent stem cells derived from bone marrow cells. These multipotent stem cells have been used for tissue-engineering studies in large animal models to investigate their potential in preclinical studies.

## 5.7 Stem Cell Therapy: Clinical Trials

The first clinical trial of cell transplantation therapy was initiated in 2005 for Alzheimer's disease (AD). In this trial, ex vivo primary fibroblasts were genetically engineered to secrete nerve growth factor (NGF) transplanted into the forebrain of eight mild AD patients. Following an average of 22 months, no long-term adverse effects were observed. Moreover, an improvement in the rate of cognitive decline was suggested with the evaluation of Mini-Mental Status Examination and Alzheimer's Disease Assessment Scale-Cognitive Subcomponent. Substantial increases in cortical fluorodeoxyglucose after the treatment were also observed by serial PET scans. One of the eight patients was analysed, and it was confirmed that transplanted cells survived and produced NGF in the brain. The most important result in the trial was that the secreted NGF induced the growth of cholinergic processes in the balsa forebrain. It means that there is a possibility that introduction of NGF with transplanted cells repairs the lost neuronal network in the AD patients' brain (Fig. 5.9). Furthermore, neurotrophic factors such as NGF and BDNF seem to play an important role for neuroprotection and functional recovery. It has been shown that NSCs can express neurotrophic factors, not only BDNF but also

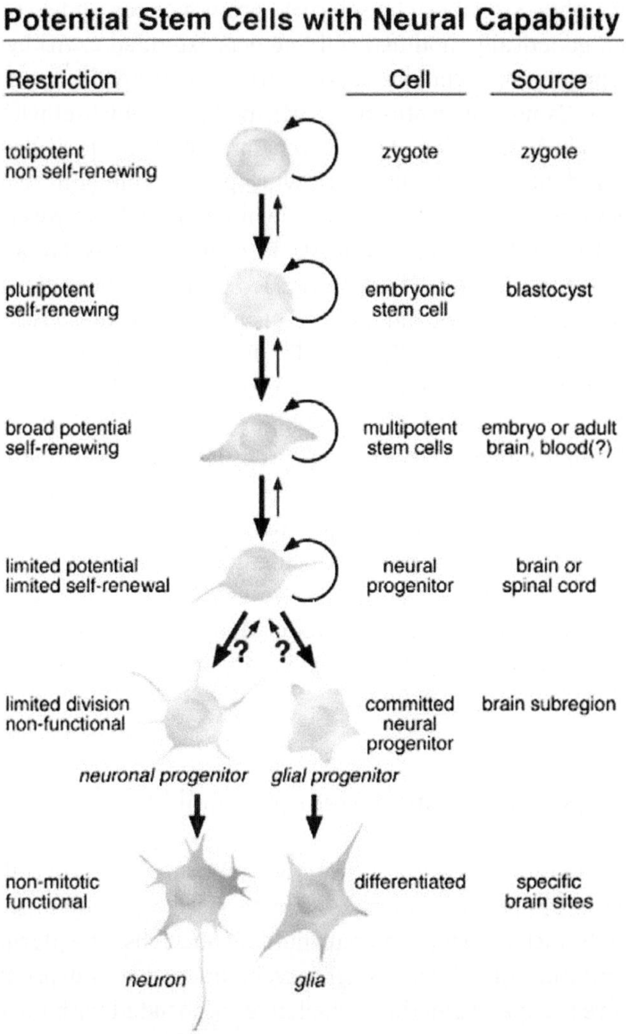


**Figure 5.9** An illustration proposing the classes of mammalian stem cells that can give rise to neurons, presented as a hierarchy beginning with the most primitive and multipotent stem cell and progressing to the most restricted. The restrictions of fate at each step and examples of sites in the body where they can be obtained are also presented. As our understanding of the true potential and nature of stem cells is still unfolding, modifications will clearly be added. For example, the small arrows pointing up suggest the potential. Reproduced with permission from Gage et al., *Science*, 287, 1433–1428 (2000).

neurotrophin-3, glial cell line-derived growth factor, and so on. The use of a genetically modified cell line was extended to AD by over-expressing human choline acetyltransferase (ChAT) gene in this NSC line. Using a neurotoxin rat AD model in which ethylcholine mustard aziridinium ion (AF64A) was intracerebroventricularly administered into the animal's brain, widespread cholinergic neuronal loss was detected and accompanied by memory deficits, resembling many of the salient features of AD. In contrast, transplantation of ChAT-positive NSCs into lesioned rats led to the recovery of learning and memory functions and induced elevated levels of acetylcholine (Ach) in cerebrospinal fluid (CSF). Further investigations have shown that the migration of the transplanted ChAT human NSCs was traced to various regions of the brain, including the cerebral cortex, hippocampus, striatum, and septum; these cells were seen to differentiate into neurons and astrocytes. From these studies, it has been shown that memory deficits and complex learning impairments are corrected by transplantation of human NSCs over-expressing ChAT in the brains of AF64A-cholinotoxin-induced AD rat model. In ALS, it may be possible to repopulate lost corticospinal and lower motor neurons by transplanting stem cells or stimulating native progenitor populations.

## 5.8 Induced Pluripotent Stem (iPS) Cell Therapy

A new generation of methods to provide pluripotent stem cells is in the process of being established. The cells are multipotent somatic stem cells, including induced pluripotent stem cells. The pluripotent differentiation of ES cells itself is very attractive and promising, but there are many bioethical challenges associated with the origin of hES cells. Scientists have looked for a breakthrough in hES cell research, providing an alternative strategy to cell replacement therapy. Induced pluripotent stem (iPS) cells are pluripotent stem cells directly reprogrammed from cultured mouse fibroblasts by introducing Oct3/4, Sox2, c-Myc, and Klf4 (Fig. 5.10). The cells obtained using this technology have pluripotentiality comparable to ES cells and can be derived from the somatic cells of patients. This advantage allows the ethical issues and immunological rejection

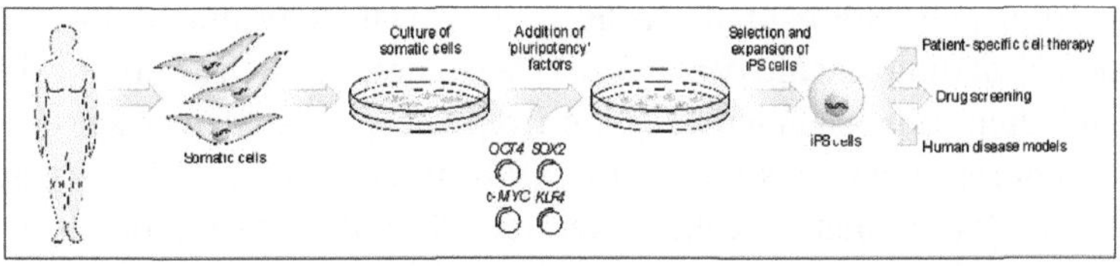


**Figure 5.10** Applications of iPS cells. To generate iPS cells, fibroblasts (or another type of adult somatic cells) are transduced with retroviruses encoding four pluripotency factors (SOX2, KLF4, c-MYC, and OCT4). Fully reprogrammed iPS cells have similar properties to ES cells. They are competent to form teratomas on injection into mice and are capable of generating progeny. A patient's cells can be used to derive iPS cells, which can then be induced to undergo differentiation into various types of somatic cells, all with the same genetic information as the patient. For example, dopaminergic neurons could be generated from the cells of a patient with Parkinson's disease and then transplanted to replace those neurons that have been lost. These differentiated cells can also be used in disease models for studying the molecular basis of a broad range of human diseases that are otherwise difficult to study (for instance, those that affect brain cells) and for screening the efficacy and safety of drug candidates for treating these diseases. Reproduced with permission from Yamanaka, *Nature*, 465, 704–712 (2010).

associated with ES cells to be avoided, and might be a clinically useful source for cell replacement therapies. Currently iPS cells can be induced from humans, mice, rats, macaque monkeys, and so on, and a method to differentiate a commercial human iPS cell line, namely IMR90 clone 4, into DA neuron progenitors is available. Transplantation of these progenitor cells into a 6-OHDA-treated rat showed long-term survival of the cells. They differentiated into DA neurons and integrated into the surrounding tissue. On the other hand, many nestin-positive tumor-like cells were found at the transplanted site. Therefore, methods to select the appropriate population of specific lineage cells are critical for iPS cell replacement therapy. Recent findings have shown that secondary neurospheres (SNSs) generated from various mouse iPS cells showed their neural differentiation capacity and teratoma formation after transplantation into the brain of immmunodeficient NOD/SCID (nonobese diabetic severe combined immunodeficient) mice. It has also been shown that the source of somatic cells for the generation of iPS cells is a crucial determinant for the potential tumorigenicity of iPS-derived neural stem/progenitor cells and their tumorigenicity results from the persistent presence of undifferentiated cells within the SNSs. Interestingly, SNSs derived from c-Myc minus iPS cells, generated without drug selection, have shown robust tumorigenesis, in spite of their potential to contribute adult chimeric mice without tumor formation. Furthermore, neuroscientists have examined whether the transplantation of non-tumorigenic Nanog-iPS-derived SNSs into mouse spinal cord injury (SCI) model could promote locomotor function recovery. As a result, properly pre-evaluated iPS clone-derived neural stem/progenitor cells may overcome the problem of high tumorigenicity of iPS cells. A combinational method with iPS cell replacement therapy and gene therapy may induce new therapy. Patient-specific iPS cells have been developed for PD due to one-point mutation in a-synuclein. The point mutation was repaired by zinc finger nuclease-mediated genome editing. The repaired human iPS cells differentiated into functional DA neurons, which bring out another advantage of iPS cells that can be available as a model for each patient, thus promoting the possibility of customized cell transplantation therapy. Furthermore, iPS cells can provide a living cell model with the potential to study early molecular changes in the cells, in which the change finally results in neurodegeneration.

Japan is one of the major players in stem cell biology and related fields. One of the reasons is the noted work that originated from the laboratory of Shinya Yamanaka, with the first report of iPS cells in 2006, and the compelling nature of the need in this country. On some reported studies, the ratio of the patients with neurodegenerative diseases, such as ALS, PD, and Alzheimer's disease, has been increasing in Japan. In spite of the fact, cell transplantation therapy has not been applied due basically to ethical problems. In June 2009, the Ministry of Health, Labour and Welfare in Japan provided the first "Guidelines on clinical research using human stem cells." Later, new guidelines were provided for human iPS cells, which focused on producing not only functional cells and tissue but also three-dimensional organs. According to the governmental plan, the RIKEN Centre for Developmental Biology (located in Kobe), the Keio University School of Medicine, and the Kyoto University Centre

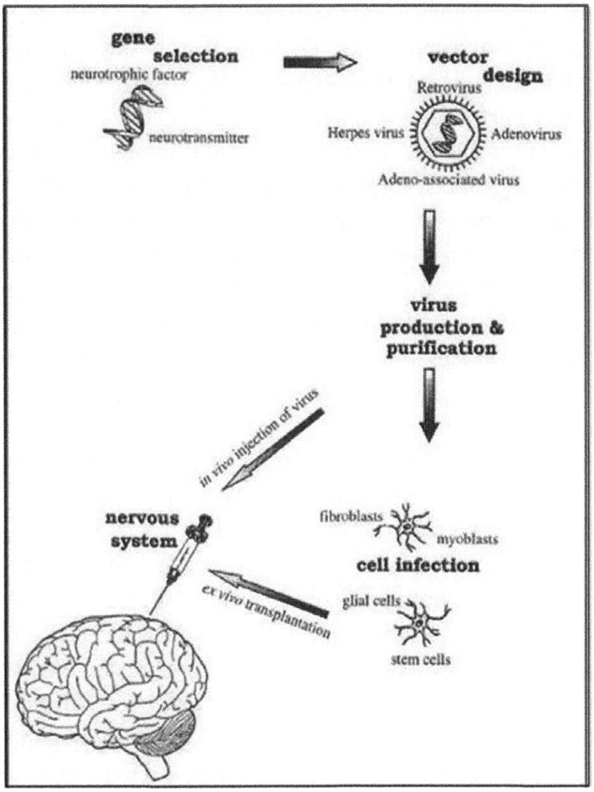


**Figure 5.11** Viruses and cell types used for experimental gene/graft therapy in the nervous system.

for iPS Cell Research and Innovation are boasting broad-spectrum studies of stem cells and iPS cells.

## 5.9 Gene Therapy and Future Challenges

Gene therapy aims at treating disease by genetically modifying cells that are either directly functionally impaired or capable of relieving the disease symptoms (Fig. 5.11). The methods are roughly separated into two groups, in vivo gene therapy and ex vivo gene therapy. The former is the direct genetic modification of cells inside the body and comprise chemical and physical methods, such as gene gun or electroporation. The latter is based on the genetic modification of cells maintained in culture prior to implantation in the patient. Particularly over the last 10 years, adeno-associated virus (AAV) has been the predominant choice for central or peripheral nervous system focused clinical trials, with 20 trials listed in 2010. The viral vector therapy takes advantage of the ability of viruses to deliver their genetic material to target cells. Cells tend to uptake materials inside during cell division, but the maturely differentiated cells, including neurons, usually are postmitiotic. So this approach utilizes the ability of infection. The other advantage is to induce long-term transgene expression. For biosafety, viral vectors are engineered from wild-type viruses by ablating the genes for replication from their genome to limit the risk of producing replication-competent viral particles. Therefore, the virus vectors are able to infect target cells and transfer their genetic material into the nucleus, but they are unable to replicate themselves in the host cells. As this viral gene therapy method may directly modify the genomes of patients because of their ability of infection, clinical trials of this therapy are currently focusing on the possibility of tumorgenicity. Several types of vectors have been developed that differ in their packaging capacity, tropism, and immunogenicity.

Lentiviruses are enveloped viruses from the Retroviridae family. Lentivectors were developed from primate lentiviruses, such as the wild-type human immunodeficiency virus type 1 (HIV-1) and nonprimate lentiviruses, such as the equine infectious anemia virus (EIAV). The lentivector has the maximal packaging capacity of 18 kb, but the most efficient packaging is obtained with genomes in the range of 6–9 kb. Lentivectors have the ability to integrate into the host cell genome and lead to stable transgene expression. This ability is very effective for ex vivo gene therapy applications, because it means that the transfected cell line or stem cells can be stably transduced and that the stability also can keep time to characterize expression of transgene prior to implantation. This property has also the risk of insertional mutagenesis, because the integration occurs at random sites. It is the biosafety for lentivectors to be considered for in vivo gene therapy. However, neuroscientists used Cdkn2a-/- mice and studied hematopoietic stem cells from these tumor-prone mice to assess the oncogenicity of prototypical lentiviral vectors. The lentiviral vectors did not affect the tumorigenesis, despite the higher integration load and robust expression of lentiviral vectors in all hematopoietic lineages. The clinical trial using lentivectors for PD patients did not report any evidence of tumorigenicity yet.

Vectors derived from AAV are the most frequent type of vectors used in clinical trials for CNS disease. AAV are small nonenveloped viruses of the Parvoviridae family. The 4.7 kb AAV genome is composed of single-stranded DNA encoding four proteins essential for replication and packaging, and three capsid proteins surrounded by two inverted terminal repeats. As AAVs are considered non-pathogenic in humans, and their capsid proteins induce only mild immune reactions, they are prime candidates for gene therapy. Viral vectors have been derived from wild-type AAVs by the deletion of all the viral sequences except the inverted terminal repeats. Moreover, AAV vectors cannot express their own viral proteins, which reduce their immunogenicity (Fig. 5.12).

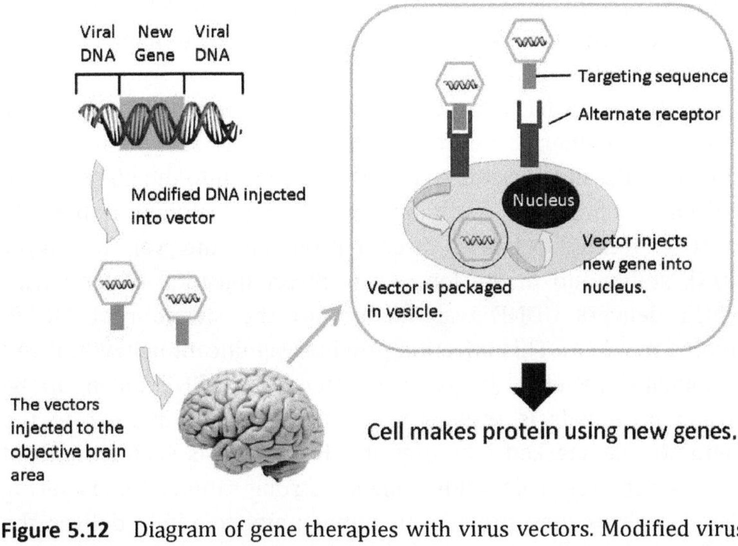


**Figure 5.12** Diagram of gene therapies with virus vectors. Modified virus vectors containing targeting capsid sequences bind alternate cell surface receptors to expand viral tropism.

AAV vector particles can efficiently infect a broad range of cells, including postmitotic cells, and display a high neuronal tropism. The viruses enter the host cell via receptor-mediated endocytosis, and they are translocated to the nucleus where their genome is converted into double-stranded DNA. Wild-type AAVs preferentially integrate to the human genome, and recombinant AAV vectors from stable episomal concatemers in the absence of the replication and packaging protein. The episomal AAV genomes provide long-term, over 1 year, transgene expression in postmitotic cells. By the above properties, AAV vectors can be ideal vectors to deliver and express genes, particularly in the CNS. The limitation of packaging of AAV vectors is about 4.7 kb, and the small range precludes the integration of large genes, or multiple expression cassettes.

There are some strategies with gene therapy to compensate the function of DA neurons in PD patients. The gene candidates are tyrosine hydroxylase (TH), aromatic amino acid decarboxylase (AADC), and GTP-cyclohydrolase-1 (GCH-1). They are enzymes to synthesize DA from tyrosine. The expression of those cells with the virus increase striatal DA in 6-OHDA lesioned rats and the therapy corrects motor deficits due to the treatment. Injection of a mixture of those three separate AAV vectors expressing TH, AADC, and GCH-1, respectively, improved manual dexterity in the putamen of MPTP-treated cynomolgus macaque monkeys.

As above, GDNF appears to have the capacity to protect or rescue dopaminergic neurons. The effect was shown in in vivo models of PD and direct implantation of GENF into the nigrostriatal system demonstrated both behavioral and histological benefits in MPTP-treated primates after a prolonged interval. To supply GDNF stably and in the long term, direct injection of lentivirus, which delivers GDNF, was made into the striatum of MPTP-treated monkeys. This injection provides significant behavioral and histological benefits. It was suggested that GDNF taken up by striatal terminals is transferred in a retrograde manner to the nigra so that marked increases in TH staining is seen in both of these structures. This study shows a strong rationale considering that lentivirus may provide an opportunity to safely deliver the trophic factor to the striatum of PD patients. Preclinical studies showed that intrastriatal injections of neurturin (a close homologue of GDNF) expressing AAV2 vector protect nigral neurons from

6-OHDA-induced degeneration and preserve animal motor behavior. Recent studies have shown that injection of AAV2 vector encoding neurturin into the striatum and SN into MPTP-treated monkeys significantly improved motor functions and the effect lasted over 10 months. The bilateral intraputaminal injection of the AAV2-neurturin vector was evaluated for safety and efficacy in an open-label phase I clinical trial. Twelve patients with diagnosis of PD received bilateral, stereotactic, intraputaminal injections of AAV2-neurturin. The patients were separated into two groups. The first six patients received a low amount of the virus vectors and the other group were injected with 5 times the amount of the vectors. The extensive safety of the vector in all patients revealed no clinically significant adverse events in 1 year. There was no difference between the low-dose group and the high-dose group in UPDRS motor score, but improvement was found in bradykinesia, rigidity tremors, and postural instability in both groups. However, the double-blind randomized phase II clinical study that followed with 58 PD patients did not show any significant beneficial effects between the control group of patients who received sham surgery and the virus-injected group.

In ALS, the latest research study based on gene therapy was on transgenic mice expressing mutant superoxide dismutase (SOD1). In this study, a gene called VEGF, which makes the endothelial growth factor protein, was injected into various different muscles, and it was found that it slowed the progression of ALS by 30% (Fig. 5.13).

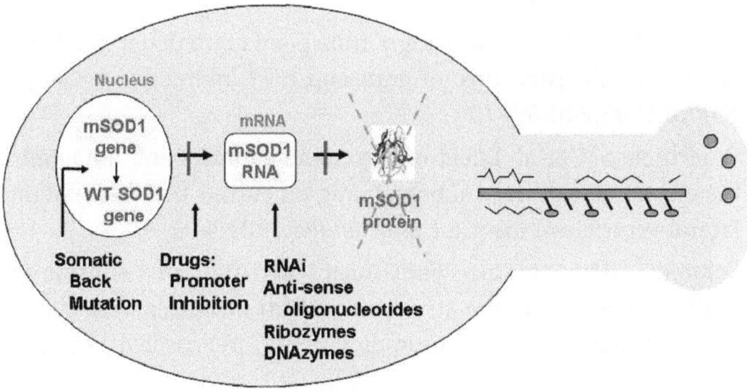


**Figure 5.13** The most proximal treatment for SOD1-related ALS is to turn off the sick gene.

In summary, advances in gene transfer techniques coupled with new insights into molecular pathology have opened promising avenues for gene therapy aimed at halting disease progression. Non-viral preparations and recombinant adenoviruses, adeno-associated viruses, herpesviruses, and lentiviruses may ultimately transduce sufficient numbers of cerebral, brainstem, and spinal cord neurons for therapeutic applications. This could be accomplished by direct injection, transduction of lower motor neurons via retrograde transport after intramuscular injection, or cell-based therapies. The challenge ahead is to translate these basic science breakthroughs into workable clinical practice.

## Further Reading


1. Perlow MJ et al. Brain grafts reduce motor abnormalities produced by destruction of nigro-striatal dopamine system. *Science* 1979;204:643–647.
2. Bjöklund A and Stenevi U. Reconstruction of the nigrostiriatal dopamine pathway by intracerebralnigral transplants. *Brain Res* 1979;177:555–560.
3. Bakay REA et al. Preliminary report on the use of fetal tissue transplantation to correct MPTP-induced Parkinson-like syndrome in primates. *Appl Neurophysiol* 1985;48:358–361.
4. Bakay REA et al. Biochemical and behaviral correction of MPTP Parkison-like syndrome by fetal cell transplantation. *Ann NY Acad Sci* 1987;495:623–638.
5. Mahalik TJ et al. Substantianigra transplants into denervated striatum of the rat: ultrastructure of graft and host interconnections. *J Comp Neurol* 1985;240:60–70.
6. Wuerthele SM et al. Effect of dopamine agonists and antagonists on the electrical activity of substantianigra neurons transplanted into the lateral ventricle of the rat. *Exp Brain Res* 1981;44:1–10.
7. Schmidt RH et al. Functional activity of substantianigra grafts reinnervating the striatum: neurotransmitter metabolism and [14C]2-deoxy-D-glucose autoradiography. *J Neurochem* 1982;38:737–748.
8. Björklund A et al. Reinnervation of the denervated striatum by substantianigra transplants: functional consequences as revealed by

pharmacological and sensorimotor testing. *Brain Res* 1980;199:307–333.

9. Dunnett SB et al. Graft-derived recovery from 6-OHDA lesions: specificity of ventral mesencephalic graft tissues. *Exp. Brain Res* 1988;71:411–424.
10. Backlund EO et al. Transplantation of adrenal medullary tissue to striatum in parkinsonism. First clinical trials. *J Neurosurg* 1985;62:169–173.
11. Lindvall O et al. Transplantation in Parkinson's disease: two cases of adrenal medullary grafts to the putamen. *Ann Neurol* 1987;22:457–468.
12. Madrazo I et al. Open microsurgical autograft of adrenal medulla to the right caudate nucleus in two patients with intractable Parkinson's disease. *N Engl J Med* 1987;316:831–834.
13. Goetz CG et al. Multicenter study of autologous adrenal medullary transplantation to the corpus striatum in patients with advanced Parkinson's disease. *N Engl J Med* 1989;320:337–341.
14. Peterson DI et al. Autopsy findings in a patient who had an adrenal-to-brain transplant for Parkinson's disease. *Neurology* 1989;39:235–238.
15. Hurtig H. Postmortem analysis of adrenal-medulla-to-caudate autograft in a patient with Parkinson's disease. *Ann Neurol* 1989;25:607–614.
16. Bohn MC et al. Adrenal medulla grafts enhance recovery of striatal dopaminergic fibers. *Science* 1987;237:913–916.
17. Fiandaca MS et al. Adrenal medullary autografts into the basal ganglia of Cebus monkeys: injury-induced regeneration. *Exp Neurol* 1988;102:76–91.
18. Brundin P. Behavioural effects of human fetal dopamine neurons grafted in a rat model of Parkinson's disease. *Exp Brain Res* 1986;65:235–240.
19. Strömberg I et al. Intracerebralxenografts of human mesencephalic tissue into athymic rats: immunochemical and in vivo electrochemical studies. *Proc Natl Acad Sci USA* 1988;85:8331–8334.
20. Lindvall O et al. Fetal dopamine-rich mesencephalic grafts in Parkinson's disease. *Lancet* 1988;332:1483–1484.
21. Lindvall O. Grafts of Fetal Dopamine Neurons Survive and Improve Motor Function in Parikinson's Disease. *Science.* 1990;247:574–577.

22. Spencer DD et al. Unilateral transplantation of human fetalmesencephalic tissue into the caudate nucleus of patients with Parkinson's disease. *N Engl J Med* 1992;327:1541–1548.
23. Freed CR et al. Survival of implanted fetal dopamine cells and neurologic improvement 12 to 46 months after transplantation for Parkinson's disease. *N Engl J Med* 1992;327:1549–1555.
24. Defer GL et al. Long-term outcome of unilaterally transplanted parkinsonian patients. I. Clinical approach. *Brain* 1996;119 (Pt 1):41–50.
25. Freed CR et al. Transplantation of embryonic dopamine neurons for severe Parkinson's disease. *N Engl J Med* 2001;344:710–719.
26. Mendez I et al. Cell type analysis of functional fetal dopamine cell suspension transplants in the striatum and substantianigra of patients with Parkinson's disease. *Brain* 2005;128:1498–1510.
27. Wenning GK et al. Short- and long-term survival and function of unilateral intrastriatal dopaminergic grafts in Parkinson's disease. *Ann Neurol* 1997;42:95–107.
28. Hagell P et al. Sequential bilateral transplantation in Parkinson's disease. Effects of the second graft. *Brain.* 1999;122:1121–1132.
29. Apostolides C et al. Glial cell line-derived neurotrophic factor improves intrastriatal graft survival of stored dopaminergic cells. *Neuroscience* 1998;83:363–372.
30. Mendez I et al. Enhancement of survival of stored dopaminergic cells and promotion of graft survival by exposure of human fetal nigral tissue to glial cell line-derived neurotrophic factor in patients with Parkinson's disease. *J Neurosurg* 2000;92:863–869.
31. Opacka-Jeffry J et al. GDNF protects against 6-OHDA nigrostriatallesion: in vivo study with microdialysis and PET. *Neuroreport* 1995;7:348–352.
32. Nikkahah G et al. Improved graft survival and striatal reinnervation by microtransplantation of fetalnigral cell suspensions in the rat Parkinson's model. *Brain Res* 1994;633:133–143.
33. Mendez I et al. Reconstruction of the nigrostriatal pathway by simultaneous intrastriatal and intranigral dopaminergic transplants. *J Neurosci* 1996;16:7216–7227.
34. Cheramy A et al. Dendritic release of dopamine in the substantianigra. *Nature* 1981;289:537–542.
35. Ruffieux A, Schultz W. Dopaminergic activation of reticulata neurones in the substantianigra. *Nature* 1980;285:40–241.

36. Martin LP, Waszczak BL. D1 agonist-induced excitation of substantianigra pars reticulata neurons: mediation by D1 receptors on striatonigral terminals via a pertussis toxin-sensitive coupling pathway. *J Neurosci* 1994;14:4494–4506.
37. Mendez I. et al. Simultaneous intrastriatal and intranigralfetal dopaminergic grafts in patients with Parkinson's disease: a pilot study. *J Neurosurg* 2002;96:589–596.
38. Hauser RA. Long-term evaluation of bilateral fetalnigral transplantation in Parkinson disease. *Arch Neurol* 1999;56:179–187.
39. Hagell P et al. Dyskinesias following neural transplantation in Parkinson's disease. *Nat Neurosci* 2002;5:627–328.
40. Zhao S et al. Generation of embryonic stem cells and transgenic mice expressing green fluorescence protein in midbrain dopaminergic neurons. *Eur J Neurosci* 2005;25:6467–6477.
41. Bolam JP et al. Synaptic input and local output of dopaminergic neurons in grafts that functionally reinnervate the host neostriatum. *Exp Brain Res* 1987;68:131–146.
42. Mahalik TJ et al. Specific outgrowth from neurons of ventral mesencephalic grafts to the catecholamine-depleted striatum of adult hosts. *Exp Neurol* 1991;113:18–27.
43. Karschin C et al. IRK(1-3) and GIRK(1-4) inwardly rectifying K+ channel mRNAs are differentially expressed in the adult rat brain. *J Neurosci* 1996;16:3559–3570.
44. Parent A et al. Calcium-binding proteins in primate basal ganglia. *Neurosci Res* 1996;25:309–334.
45. Chung S et al. The homeodomain transcription factor Pitx3 facilitates differentiation of mouse embryonic stem cells into AHD2-expressing dopaminergic neurons. *Mol Cell Neurosci* 2005;28:241–252.
46. Thompson L et al. Identification of dopaminergic neurons of nigral and ventral tegmental area subtypes in grafts of fetal ventral mesencephalon based on cell morphology, protein expression, and efferent projections. *J Neurosci* 2005;25:6467–6477.
47. Thompson L et al. Non-dopaminergic neurons in ventral mesencephalic transplants make widespread axonal connections in the host brain. *Exp Neurol* 2008;213:220–228.
48. Carlsson T et al. Serotonin neuron transplants exacerbate L-DOPA-induced dyskinesias in a rat model of Parkinson's disease. *J Neurosci* 2007;27:8011–8022.

49. Piccini P. Dopamine release from nigral transplants visualized in vivo in a Parkinson's patient. *Nat Neurosci* 1999;2:1137–1140.
50. Thomson JA et al. Embryonic stem cell lines derived from human blastocysts. *Science* 1998:282;1145–1147.
51. Evans MJ and Kaufman MH. Establishment in culture of pluripotential cells from mouse embryos. *Nature* 1981;292:154–156.
52. Martin GR. Isolation of a pluripotent cell line from early mouse embryos cultured in medium conditioned by teratocarcinoma stem cells. *Proc Natl Acad Sci USA* 1981;78:7634–7638.
53. Lee S-H et al. Efficient generation of midbrain and hindbrain neurons from mouse embryonic stem cells. *Nat. Biotechnol.* 2000;18:675–679.
54. Kim J-H et al. Dopamine neurons derived from embryonic stem cells function in an animal model of Parkinson's disease. *Nature* 2002;418:50–56.
55. Kawasaki H et al. Generation of dopaminergic neurons and pigmented epithelia from primate ES cells by stromal cell-derived inducing activity. *Proc Natl Acad Sci USA* 2002;99:1580–1585.
56. Li XJ et al. Specification of motoneurons from human embryonic stem cells. *Nature Biotechnol* 2005;23:215–221.
57. Perrier AL et al. Derivation of midbrain dopamine neurons from human embryonic stem cells. *Proc Natl Acad Sci USA* 2004;101:12543–12548.
58. Roy NS et al. Functional engraftment of human ES cell-derived dopaminergic neurons enriched by coculture with telomerase-immortalized midbrain astrocytes. *Nature Med* 2006;12:1259–1268.
59. Elkabetz Y et al. Human ES cell-derived neural rosettes reveal a functionally distinct early neural stem cell stage. *Genes Dev* 2008;22:152–165(.
60. Kriks S et al. Dopamine neurons derived from human ES cells efficiently engraft in animal models of Parkinson's disease. *Nature* 2011;480:547–553.
61. Roelink H et al. Floor plate and motor neuron induction by vhh-1, a vertebrate homolog of hedgehog expressed by the notochord. *Cell* 1994;76:761–775.
62. Roy NS et al. Functional engraftment of human ES cell-derived dopaminergic neurons enriched by coculture with telomerase-immortalized midbrain astrocytes. *Nature Med* 2006;12:1259–1268.

63. Ferrari D, Sanchez-Pernaute R, Lee H, Studer L and Isacson O. Transplanted dopamine neurons derived from primate ES cells preferentially innervate DARPP- 32 striatal progenitors within the graft. *Eur J Neurosci* 2006;24:1885–1896.
64. Doi D et al. Prolonged maturation culture favors a reduction in the tumorigenicity and the dopaminergic function of human ESC-derived neural cells in a primate model of Parkinson's disease. *Stem Cells* 2012;30:935–945.
65. Scwarltz SD et al. Embryonic stem cell trials for macular degeneration: a preliminary report. *Lancet* 2012;379:713–720.
66. Ambati J and Fowler BJ. Mechanisms of age-related macular degeneration. *Neuron* 2012;75:26–39.
67. Gage FH. Mammalian neural stem cells. *Science* 2000;287:1433–1428.
68. Studer et al. Transplantation of expanded mesencephalic precursors leads to recovery in parkinsonian rats. *Nat Neurosci* 1998;1:290–295.
69. Wagner J et al. Induction of a midbrain dopaminergic phenotype in Nurr1-overexpressing neural stem cells by type 1 astrocytes. *Nat Biotechnol* 1999;17:653–659.
70. Xiao Q et al. Distribution of messenger RNAs for the orphan nuclear receptors Nurr1 and Nur77 (NGFI-B) in adult rat brain using in situ hybridization. *Neuroscience* 1996;75:221–230.
71. Zetterström RH et al. Dopamine neuron agenesis in Nurr1-deficient mice. *Science* 1997;267:248–250.
72. Buervenich S et al. NURR1 mutations in cases of schizophrenia and manic-depressive disorder. *Am. J. Med. Genet.* 2000;96:808–813.
73. Carmine A. NURR1 promoter polymorphisms: Parkinson's disease, schizophrenia, and personality traits. *Am J Med Genet B Neuropsychiatr Genet* 2003;120B:51–57.
74. Kim HJ et al. Control of neurogenesis and tyrosine hydroxylase expression in neural progenitor cells through bHLH proteins and Nurr1. *Exp Neurol* 2007;203:394–405.
75. Sakurada K et al. Nurr1, an orphan nuclear receptor, is a transcriptional activator of endogenous tyrosine hydroxylase in neural progenitor cells derived from the adult brain. *Development* 1999;126:4017–4026.
76. Courtois ET et al. In vitro and in vivo enhanced generation of human A9 dopamine neurons from neural stem cells by Bcl-XL. *J Biol Chem* 2010;285:9881–9897.

77. Daadi MM and Weiss S. Generation of tyrosine hydroxylase-producing neurons from precursors of the embryonic and adult forebrain. *J Neurosci* 1999;19:4484–4497.
78. Nakatomi H et al. Regeneration of hippocampal pyramidal neurons after ischemic brain injury by recruitment of endogenous neural progenitors. *Cell* 2002;110:429–441.
79. Lie DC et al. The adult substantianigra contains progenitor cells with neurogenic potential. *J. Neurosci.* 2002;22:6639–6649.
80. Suzuki H et al. Neurospheres induced from bone marrow stromal cells are multipotent for differentiation into neuron, astrocyte, and oligodendrocyte phenotypes. *Biochem. Biophys. Res. Commun.* 2004;322:918–922.
81. Jiang Y et al. Neuroectodermal differentiation from mouse multipotent adult progenitor cells. *Proc Natl Acad Sci USA* 2003;100(Suppl. 1):11854–11860.
82. Toma JG et al. Isolation and characterizationof multipotent skin-derived precursors from human skin. *Stem Cells* 2005;23:727–737.
83. Gronthos S et al. Postnatal human dental pulp stem cells (DPSCs) in vitro and in vivo. *Proc Natl Acad Sci USA* 2000;97:13625–13630.
84. Sonoyama W et al. Characterization of the apical papilla and its residing stem cells from human immature permanent teeth: a pilot study. *J Endod* 2008;34:166–171.
85. Holtzman DM. Alzheimer's disease: Moving towards a vaccine. *Nature* 2008;454:418–420.
86. Tuszynski MH et al. A phase 1 clinical trial of nerve growth factor gene therapy for Alzheimer disease. *Nat Med* 2005;11:551–555.
87. Blurton-Jones M et al. Neural stem cells improve cognition via BDNF in a transgenic model of Alzheimer disease. *Proc Natl Acad Sci USA* 2009;105:13594–13599.
88. Wu S et al. Neural stem cells improve learning and memory in rats with Alzheimer's disease. *Pathobiology* 2008;75:186–194.
89. Srivastava N et al. Long-term functional restoration by neural progenitor cell transplantation in rat model of cognitive dysfunction: co-transplantation with olfactory ensheathing cells for neurotrophic factor support. *Int J Dev Neurosci* 2009;27:103–110.
90. Schäbitz WR et al. Intravenous brain-derived neurotrophic factor reduces infarct size and counterregulatesBax and Bcl-2 expression after temporary focal cerebral ischemia. *Stroke* 2000;31:2212–2217.

91. Park D et al. Human neural stem cells over-expressing choline acetyltransferase restore cognition in rat model of cognitive dysfunction. *Exp Neurol* 2012;234:521–526.
92. Takahashi K and Yamanaka S. Induction of Pluripotent Stem cells from Mouse Embryonic and Adult Fibroblast Cultures by Defined Facors. *Cell* 2006;126:663–676.
93. Yamanaka S and Blau HM. Nuclear reprogramming to a pluripotent state by three approaches. *Nature* 2010;465:704–712.
94. Cai J et al. Dopaminergic Neurons Derived from Human Induced Pluripotent Stem Cells Survive and Integrate into 6-OHDA-Lesioned Rats. *Stem Cells Dev* 2010;19:1017–1023.
95. Nori et al. Grafted human-induced pluripotent stem-cell-derived neurospheres promote motor function recovery after spinal cord injur in mice. *Proc Natl Acad Sci USA* 2011;108:16825–16830.
96. Soldner F et al. Generation of isogenic pluripotent stem cells differing exclusively at two early onset Parkinson point mutations. *Cell* 2011;146:318–331.
97. Nakajima F Human leukocyte antigen matching estimations in a hypothetical bank of human embryonic stem cell lines in the Japanese population for use in cell transplantation therapy. *Stem Cells* 2007;25:983–985.
98. Lim ST et al. Viral vectors for neurotrophic factor delivery: A gene therapy approach for neurodegenerative disease of the CNS. *Pharmacol Res* 2010;61:14–26.
99. Naldini L et al. In vivo gene delivery and stable transduction of nondividing cells by a lentiviral vector. *Science* 1996;272:263–267.
100. Zufferey R et al. Multiply attenuated lentiviral vector achieves efficient gene delivery in vivo. *Nat Biotechnol* 1997;15;871–875.
101. Olsen JC. Gene transfer vectors derived from equine infectious anemiavirus. *Gene Ther* 1998;5:1481–1487.
102. Kumar M et al. Systematic determination of the packaging limit of lentiviral vectors. *Hum Gene Ther* 2001;12:1893–1905.
103. Montini E et al. Hematopoietic stem cell gene transfer in a tumor-prone mouse model uncovers low genotoxicity of lentiviral vector integration. *Nat Biotechnol* 2006;24:687–696.
104. Büning H et al. Recent developments in adeno-associated virus vector technology. *J Gene Med* 2008;10:717–733.

105. Paterna JC et al. Transduction profiles of recombinant adeno-associated virus vectors derived from serotypes 2 and 5 in the nigrostriatal system of rats. *J Virol* 2004;78:6808–6817.
106. Shen Y et al. Triple transduction with adeno-associated virus vectors expressing tyrosine hydroxylase, aromatic-L-amino-acid decarboxylase, and GTP cyclohydrolase I for gene therapy of Parkinson's disease. *Hum Gene Ther* 2000;11:1509–1519.
107. Sun M et al. Correction of a rat model of Parkinson's disease by coexpression of tyrosine hydroxylase and aromatic amino acid decarboxylase from a helper virus-free herpes simplex virus type 1 vector. *Hum Gene Ther* 2003;14:415–424.
108. Muramatsu S et al. Behavioral recovery in a primate model of Parkinson's disease by triple transduction of striatal cells with adeno-associated viral vectors expressing dopamine-synthesizing enzymes. *Hum Gene Ther* 2002;13:345–354.
109. Gash DM. Morphologicalandfunctionaleffectsofintranigrallyadministered GDNF in normal rhesusmonkeys. *J Clin Neuroscience* 1995; 363:345–358.
110. Gash DM. Functional recovery in parkinsonian monkeys treated with GDNF. *Nature* 1996;380:352–355.
111. Kordower JH et al. Neurodegeneration prevented by lentiviral vector delivery of GDNF in primate models of Parkinson's disease. *Science* 2000;290:767–773.
112. Kordower JH et al. Delivery of neurturin by AAV2 (CERE-120)-mediated gene transfer provides structural and functional neuroprotection and neurorestoration in MPTP-treated monkeys. *Ann Neurol* 2006;60:706–715.
113. Marks WJ Jr et al. Safety and tolerability of intraputaminal delivery of CERE-120 (adeno-associated virus serotype 2-neurturin) to patients with idiopathic Parkinson's disease: an open-label, phase I trial. *Lancet Neurol* 2008;7:400–408.
114. Marks WJ Jr et al. Gene delivery of AAV2-neurturin for Parkinson's disease: a double-blind, randomised, controlled trial. *Lancet Neurol.* 2010;9:1164–1172.
115. Bartus RT et al. Bioactivity of AAV2-neurturin gene therapy (CERE-120): differences between Parkinson's disease and nonhuman primate brains.
116. Tyler CM and Federoff HJ. CNS gene therapy and a nexus of complexity: systems and biology at a crossroads. *Cell Transplant* 2006;15:267–273.

117. Kim SU. Genetically engineered human neural stem cells for brain repair in neurological diseases. *Brain Dev* 2007;29:193–201.
118. Bruijn LI, Cudkowicz M. Therapeutic targets for amyotrophic lateral sclerosis: current treatments and prospects for more effective therapies. *Expert Rev Neurother* 2006;6:417–228.
119. Brooks BR. Managing amyotrophic lateral sclerosis: slowing disease progression and improving patient quality of life. *Ann Neurol* 2009;65(suppl1):S17–23
120. Joseph M Alisky and Beverly L Davidson. *Human Gene Therapy*. November 2000;11(17):2315–2329. doi:10.1089/104303400750038435.

# List of Abbreviations

| | |
|---|---|
| ALS | amyotrophic lateral sclerosis |
| BBB | blood–brain barrier |
| ALSFRS | ALS Functional Rating Scale |
| Cho | choline |
| Cr | creatine |
| CS | corticospinal tract |
| DTI | diffusion tensor imaging |
| FA | fractional anisotropy |
| FLAIR | fluid-attenuated inversion recovery |
| fMRI | functional MR imaging |
| FTD | frontotemporal dementia |
| FUS/TLS | fused in sarcoma/translocated in liposarcoma gene |
| GM | gray matter |
| 1H-MR spectroscopy | proton MR spectroscopy |
| L | left |
| MD | mean diffusivity |
| mIns | myo-inositol |
| NAA | N-acetylaspartate |
| PD | proton density |
| R | right |
| SOD1 | superoxide dismutase 1 |
| TDP-43 | TAR DNA-binding protein gene |
| VBM | voxel-based morphometry |
| WM | white matter |
| A$\beta$ | $\beta$-amyloid |
| AD | Alzheimer's disease |
| BMVEC | brain microvessel endothelial cells |

| | |
|---|---|
| CMC | critical micelle concentration |
| CNS | central nervous system |
| CSF | cerebrospinal fluid |
| CST | corticospinal tract |
| DTI | diffusion tensor imaging |
| EAE | experimental autoimmune encephalomyelitis |
| EPR | permeability and retention |
| HIV-1 | human immunodeficiency virus type 1 |
| GDNF | glial cell line-derived neurotrophic factor |
| GFAP | glial fibrillary acidic protein |
| MP | mononuclear phagocytes |
| MPTP | 1-methyl-4-phenyl-1, 2, 3, 6-tetrahydropyridine |
| MRI | magnetic resonance imaging |
| MRS | magnetic resonance spectroscopy |
| MRSI | magnetic resonance spectroscopic imaging |
| MS | multiple sclerosis |
| NAA | N-acetylaspartate |
| 6-OHDA | 6-hydroxydopamine |
| PD | Parkinson's disease |
| PEG | polyethylene glycol |
| PET | positron emission tomography |
| Pluronic® | poly(ethylene glycol)–b-poly(ethylene glycol)–b-poly(ethylene glycol) |
| PTD | protein-transduction domain |
| Qdots | quantum dots |
| RPE | retinal pigment epithelium |
| SCID | severe combined immunodeficiency (mouse) |
| SNpc | substantia nigra pars compacta |
| 6-OHDA | 6-hydroxydopamine |
| DA | dopamine |
| MPTP | 1,2,3,6-tetrahydropyridine |
| PET | Positron Emission Tomography |
| GDNF | glial cell line-derived neurotrophic factor |
| ES cell | embryonic stem cell |
| hES cell | human embryonic stem cell |
| UMN | Upper Motor Neurons |
| LMN | Lower Motor Neurons |
| SN | substantia nigra |

| | |
|---|---|
| AD | Alzheimer's disease |
| NGF | nerve growth factor |
| ChAT | choline acetyltransferase |
| AAV | adeno-associated virus |
| AChEIs | Acetylcholinesterase inhibitors |
| $A\beta$ Amyloid$\beta$ | A$\beta$42 One of the two most common isoforms of Amyloid-$\beta$ protein with the following Nucleotide Sequence: ASP ALA GLU PHE ARG HIS ASP SER GLY TYR GLU VAL HIS HIS GLN LYS LEU VAL PHE PHE ALA GLU ASP VAL GLY SER ASN LYS GLY ALA ILE ILE GLY LEU MET VAL GLY GLY VAL VAL ILE ALA |
| AD | Alzheimer's disease |
| ADDL | Amyloid $\beta$-Derived Diffusible Ligand |
| AgNP | Silver nanoparticle |
| AuNP | Gold nanoparticle |
| BBB | Blood brain barrier |
| C60HyFn | Nanostructures of hydrated C60 fullerene |
| CdS | Cadmium sulfate |
| CdSe | Cadmium selenide |
| CeO2 | Cerium oxide |
| CSF | Cerebrospinal fluid |
| CNS | Central nervous system |
| FDA | Food and Drug Administration of U.S. Government |
| LSPR | Localized surface plasmon resonance |
| | Lysosomes Digestive organelles in animal cells |
| NIAD-4 | A NIR Alzheimer's dye with the chemical formula [[5-(4-Hydroxyphenyl)[2,2-bithiophen]-5-yl] methylene]-propanedinitrile |
| NIR | near-infrared |
| NMDA | N-Methyl-D-aspartic acid or N-Methyl-D-aspartate |
| ORMOSIL | Organically modified silica |
| PnBCA | Poly n-butylcyanoacrylate |
| PCR | Polymerase chain reaction |
| PEG | Polyethylene glycol |
| PnBCA | Poly n- |
| ROS | Reactive oxygen |

| | |
|---|---|
| SLN | Solid lipid nanoparticles |
| STM | Scanning tunneling microscopy |
| SWCN | Single-wall carbon nanotubes |
| MPB-PE | 1,2-Dioleoyl-snglycero-3-phosphoethanolamine-N-[4-(pmaleimidophenyl) butyramide] PDP-PE MPB-PE) and pyridyldithio-propionyl-phosphoethanolamine |

# Index

acetylcholine 73, 76, 124, 145
adeno-associated virus (AAV) 128, 131, 140, 141, 145
ALSin 9
amyloid 65–67, 75, 79, 85, 144
amyloid oligomerization 65
amyloidogenesis 66
angiogenin protein 12
anterior horn cells 13, 30
antioxidant agents 75, 112
antioxidant reactions 65
atropine 100

Babinski sign 4
Betz cells 15, 30
BMAA (methylamino-L-alanine) 29–32
brain stem 1, 33, 40, 41, 44, 119
bulbar dysfunction 15

cadmium 51, 145
cell replacement therapy 102, 103, 105, 107, 111, 124–126
ceramide 88
cerebellar degeneration 19
cerium oxide 67, 145
cervical cord 43, 45
C-H2 groups 87
cholesterol ester 87, 88
chromosome 8–12, 18
CNS drug delivery 66, 70–72, 78, 92
cognitive impairment 2, 10, 57, 65, 70, 82, 91
CST 41–45
cytotoxic oxygen radicals 8, 143

dementia 6, 8, 19, 29–33, 42, 43, 57, 85, 143
dendrimers 61, 66, 67, 69, 79
desferrioxamine 74
diamondoids 67
diffuse Lewy bodies 33
DNA/RNA helicase 10
dysphagia 15

electromyography 2, 36, 39
electrophysiology 37, 47
embryonic stem ES cells 113, 114, 117, 136–138, 140, 144
EMG 2, 38, 39, 47, 52, 54
endothelial 77, 92, 93, 131, 144
eosinophilic intracytoplasmic 13

familial ALS 7–13, 143
flail leg syndrome 4
frontotemporal dementia 6, 8
FUS/TLS gene 6, 143

GABA encepha 100, 112
GDNF 108–110, 115–116, 130, 131, 135, 141, 144

gene therapy 76, 87, 96, 99, 126–131, 139–141
glial cells 45, 112, 121
glutamate receptors 30, 68
glutamatergic dysfunction 68
glycoprotein 72, 79, 91, 93, 95, 144

hES cells 114–119, 124
hexosaminidase 18
hydrogel nanoparticles 66
hyperreflexia 9, 15, 38

iPS cells 124–127

lentiviruses 128, 131
lipid 61, 68, 70, 75, 78, 79, 88, 96, 146
lipophilic 60, 74, 75
liposomes 61, 70–76, 79–81, 93
LMX1A 115

macular dystrophy 116, 118, 119
mesencephalic cells 109
mesencephalon 102, 104, 109, 112, 119, 136
microscopy 81, 83, 86, 87, 90, 92, 96, 146
midbrain 87, 112, 115, 136–138
mitochondrial genes 12
motor neuron 1–17, 30–45, 54, 63, 79, 85–111, 124
MR imaging 41–43, 90–92, 143
muscular atrophy 5–6, 15, 34
mutation 6–15, 23, 34, 121, 126, 138, 140

nanocarrier 61–63, 68, 71, 73, 75, 76, 80
nanogels 61, 65–67
nanoimaging 92, 96
Nano-N2PY 75
neuroimaging 36, 49, 50, 51, 55–58, 82, 126
neuropathological 30, 33, 36, 40
neuroprotective 16, 64–68
neurospheres 125, 138, 140
neurotoxicity 30, 64–67, 102
neurotransmitter 68, 71, 73, 133
neurotrophic factors 122
N-methyl-D-aspartat 100, 145

6-OHDA 102, 110, 119, 125, 131, 133, 135, 139, 144
oligonucleotides 66
ORMOSIL 76, 77, 145
oxidation 67

PET scans 57, 64, 82, 92, 100, 105, 111, 120, 122, 125, 128, 134, 135, 144, 145
pluronic 63, 72, 73, 80, 92, 144
polymeric micelles 72, 144
primary lateral sclerosis 6, 9, 49
primary motor cortex 1, 44–46
progressive muscular atrophy 6
protein aggregation 33

quantum dots 82, 144

radiculopathy 41
reactive oxygen intermediates (ROI) 88
riluzole 100, 101

SECARS 86–90, 92, 96
sphingolipid metabolism 88
sphingomyelin 87, 145

spinal cord 1, 15, 18, 30, 41, 55, 56, 90, 92, 93, 114, 126, 131, 140
sporadic 6, 8, 14–23, 30, 36, 51, 55, 99
sporadic ALS 6, 8, 13–17, 36, 51, 55
stem cells 77, 90, 92, 113, 114, 119, 121–129, 136–141
superoxide dismutase 1 (SOD1) 6, 7, 8, 13, 14, 25, 79, 131–132, 143
surface enhanced nanoimaging 92, 96
surface plasmon resonance 79, 80, 83, 145

transcytosis 60, 77
transgenic 34, 85–90, 109, 111, 131, 136, 139, 157
transplantation 102–107, 110–119, 122–126, 133–140

upper motor neurons 2–12, 15, 33, 35, 37, 40–41, 143
USPIO 83, 85–92, 96

VAPB genes 13
VEGF 131
voxel-based morphometry 43, 58, 143

An environmentally friendly book printed and bound in England by www.printondemand-worldwide.com

PEFC Certified

This product is from sustainably managed forests and controlled sources

www.pefc.org

PEFC

PEFC/16-33-415

This book is made of chain-of-custody materials; FSC materials for the cover and PEFC materials for the text pages.